商务话语与文化研究丛书

总主编　郭桂杭　**副总主编**　胡春雨

A Contrastive Study of Medical Promotional Discourses:

From the Perspective of Cognitive Grammar

认知语法视角下的医疗推广语篇对比研究

杨文慧　著

科学出版社

北　京

内 容 简 介

本书是对《认知语义学视角下的跨文化商务传媒语篇研究》的补充，基于认知科学视域和跨文化语言对比视角，将实证研究数据和认知模型相结合深入探讨和分析跨文化语篇中语用和认知构建。本书以认知语法为切入点，基于构式语法和词法的实证分析，诠释不同文化和语系的医疗推广语篇中转喻视点语法、语步结构中的力动态语法和情态动词的情景入场语法的意义识解和认知模型，旨在揭示英汉医疗推广语篇中跨文化认知语言差异，助力跨文化商务交际、企业出海和产品国际市场化的推广。

本书可供应用语言学、认知科学、大众传媒和商务英语专业的学者、从事产品推广和语篇制作的专业人士阅读和参考。

图书在版编目（CIP）数据

认知语法视角下的医疗推广语篇对比研究=A Contrastive Study of Medical Promotional Discourses: From the Perspective of Cognitive Grammar: 英文 / 杨文慧著. —北京：科学出版社，2024.3

（商务话语与文化研究丛书/郭桂杭总主编）

ISBN 978-7-03-078170-3

Ⅰ. ①认… Ⅱ. ①杨… Ⅲ. ①医疗保健事业–市场营销学–英语–研究 Ⅳ. ①R19

中国国家版本馆 CIP 数据核字（2024）第 053645 号

责任编辑：常春娥 / 责任校对：宁辉彩
责任印制：徐晓晨 / 封面设计：润一文化

科 学 出 版 社 出版
北京东黄城根北街 16 号
邮政编码：100717
http://www.sciencep.com
北京建宏印刷有限公司印刷
科学出版社发行　各地新华书店经销

*

2024 年 3 月第 一 版　　开本：720×1000　1/16
2024 年 3 月第一次印刷　　印张：15
字数：313 000
定价：118.00 元
（如有印装质量问题，我社负责调换）

总　　序

白 2007 年教育部批准设置商务英语本科专业全今，随着国家"一带一路"倡议的提出，我国国际贸易、国际投资等国际商务活动快速增长，设立商务英语专业的学校也得以迅猛发展，截至 2018 年，共有 367 所高校开办商务英语本科专业，探索人才培养模式，服务于国家和区域经济发展需要。商务英语在国外不作为一个独立专业，但在我国，随着国家高等教育大力发展新兴交叉学科总体战略目标的提出、人才培养需要的增加及商务英语教学实践的深入，商务英语学科理论研究日益受到国内专家学者的重视，并已经取得一些研究成果。一些论文在国内外有影响力的期刊上发表，也有若干涉及商务英语教师发展的著作相继出版。

在人才培养和学科建设方面，广东外语外贸大学国际商务英语学院也在一直努力探索开拓。继 2007 年申办商务英语本科专业之后，我们先后率先在外国语言文学一级学科下开设了商务英语研究二级硕士学位授权点和博士学位授权点，形成了完整的本科、硕士和博士人才培养体系和学科层次。商务英语研究的独特性和学科交叉性、研究内容的包容性、研究方法的多样性已突破了外国语言学及应用语言学学科的限制，它融合了语言学、经济学、管理学、社会学、教育学等多个学科类别，具有鲜明的跨学科性质。我们这次编辑出版"商务话语与文化研究丛书"，就是一种交叉学科研究的尝试。在国内学界享有盛誉的科学出版社高瞻远瞩，大力扶持商务英语研究，欣然同意出版这套丛书。丛书为国内商务英语话语与文化研究者提供一个平台，较为系统地展示国内学者在商务话语与文化领域的研究新成果，供广大同行分享。

本丛书由商务话语与商务文化两类研究话题构成，首批著作主要涉及以下话题：多模态广告话语研究、英语商业广告语篇隐性连贯的识解机制研究、社会-认知视角下 BELF（business English as a lingua franca）交际中的元语用话语研究、中美上市公司年报 MD&A（management discussion and analysis）中语言策略对比研究、转型期中国农村保险销售互动话语研究、商务会议冲突管理中的高效信息交换研究、中外会计文化对比研究、语言博弈论视角下的跨文化商务谈判互动研究、基于认知视角下的跨文化商务传媒语篇研究。本丛书的作者均为商务话语或商务文化研究领域的学者，相信本丛书的出版将进一步促进国内商务话语与文化研究的发展。

　　本丛书是一个开放的平台。鉴于商务英语研究的跨学科性质，我们希望本丛书以外国语言学及应用语言学为坚实的学科基础，旁及其他学科，研究者能在中外比较研究中、在不同视角中、在学科交叉中、在观点碰撞中去从事学术研究。欢迎广大同仁提供自己的新作，和我们一起紧扣时代需要，探索和拓展新领域，发现和研究新问题，为国家社会经济文化建设服务。

　　本丛书的出版得到广东外语外贸大学高水平学科建设项目的大力支持，也得到科学出版社编辑们的鼎力相助，在此对他们表示衷心的感谢。本丛书的首批著作是近年来广东外语外贸大学商务英语学科领域的部分研究成果，"路漫漫其修远兮，吾将上下而求索"，我们深知学术求索之艰辛，丛书中可能存在有待商榷的学术问题，敬请专家学者给予批评指正。我们也热忱欢迎同行学者不吝赐稿，为本丛书的成长壮大添砖加瓦。我们愿与国内同行一起，为商务英语学科的发展壮大而努力。

郭桂杭

2018 年 6 月于广东外语外贸大学

前　　言

　　认知语言学作为一门新兴交叉学科，将认知科学与语言学（如形式语言学和功能语言学）相结合，在约四十年中取得了丰硕的成果（如 Langacker 1987a，1991，2001，2008；Talmy 1988，2000；Croft & Cruse 2004；Kövecses 2006；Yang 2020）。本书重点关注的是认知语言的体验主义，它强调在特定的文化背景下，人类在其社会活动历程中身体和空间上的体验，认知语言的体验主义为认知语言学和跨文化研究的结合提供了基本立足点。认知语言学研究和跨文化研究都将语言或话语置于中心位置，深入研究其与文化中的潜在价值观和意识形态的关系，这类研究主要基于以下三点。第一，将语言现象与文化联系起来以便于读者了解语言在实际情境中如何运用，所以有必要将语言放在真实文化语境中进行（跨文化比较）研究。第二，考虑到语言是文化中不可或缺的一部分，对语言使用的分析不足在某种程度上会导致跨文化研究的不足。尽管不少学者在词汇或语义层面已经做了很多努力，但是从跨文化视角进行的认知和语篇研究还有待加强。第三，语言文化的差异体现于多层面的认知构架。文化价值主要是由社会、个人的认知体验通过语言选择实现的。尽管人们生活在不同的文化中，但在知识和交际经验方面却有很多相似之处。这就解释了为什么不同文化背景的人可能会使用相同的认知模式和话语进行表达，并能够识别现有的实体和概念。然而，多样的文化背景和个人经历往往会产生不同的体验，使得语篇和话语表达方式（如语法、句法和词法等）有所不同。

　　在前人研究基础上，本书以认知语法为研究视角，以中英文医疗推广语篇（医药、医疗器械和互联网线上治疗推广语篇）为研究文本，通过实证方式分析认知语法结构所涉及的转喻视点语法（Metonymic PoV Grammar）、语步结构中的力动态语法（Force Dynamic Grammar in Move Structure）以及情态动词的情景入场语法（Modal Verb Grounding Grammar），探索跨文化语篇中特定认知模式和意义构建的语法原则，以及这些语法原则与语篇中的概念表征和语言选择的关联和意义，本书也是笔者 2020 年出版的专著《认知语义学视角下的跨文化商务传媒语篇研究》在认知语法层面的延伸研究。这种在认知层面分析语言选择和语法的方式使我们可以更广泛地将语言、语用、语篇和语法现象联系起来，在认知中寻找语言表征和文化语言范式，从而丰富应用语言学和认知语言学研究的内涵和范畴。此外，本书从跨文化角度对比分析中英文医疗产品推广所构建的大众认知差异如何影响消费者的认知行为，从而为我国医药产品走向世界并在世界市场取得商务话语权提供语用、语篇方面的借鉴和研究基础。本书由七章组成。

第一章梳理相关传媒语篇研究现状和医疗推广语篇的研究基础，并介绍本书所涉及的医疗推广语篇的研究背景和研究发展状况。在第二章中，笔者提出了本书的理论依据和研究框架。在该章中，笔者不仅对认知语言学的发展进行了批判性的回顾，对当前认知语法研究理论存在的问题和缺陷提出了自己的见解，还将词项语法作为本次深入探究认知语言学和语篇分析的切入点，并对词项语法的三个研究点（词项语法中的视点、力动态和入场语法）的语法定义和分类进行了细致解读。第三章介绍当前跨文化对比研究的研究趋势以及跨文化对比研究设计。该章说明了英文语篇来源；基于实证研究和中英文医疗产品服务推广的语篇分析，针对分类筛选后的词项语法，笔者使用网页爬虫工具八爪鱼（Octopus）和语料库工具小蚂蚁（AntConc）搜索相关语法的语言表征，通过定性和定量分析来解读跨文化认知差异和认知构建模式。第四、五、六章基于第二章词项语法的研究理论，具体分析和论述了抗癌药物推广语篇中的转喻视点语法（Metonymic Point of View Grammar/Metonymic PoV Grammar）、在线医疗推广语篇语步结构中的力动态语法和医疗设备心脏支架推广语篇中的情态动词的情景入场语法，以及三章语篇分析的语料来源和不同词项语法的意义、结构、时态等所构建的认知框架和语用策略。第七章对认知语法的语用与语篇跨文化差异进行了更为深入的阐述，并探讨了认知语法在医疗推广语篇研究中的现实意义和语用策略。此外，笔者在战略思维层面对跨文化认知差异进行了诠释，分析了如何让中国医疗产品以及其他商务产品为世人认知，为实现中国产品国际化提供实证依据和语言层面的支持。最后，笔者总结了本书主要的跨文化交际发现，并对认知语言学、社会语言学和跨文化沟通研究未来的发展方向提出了自己的看法，同时对中国医疗要走向世界应如何提升营销语言策略、重构跨文化认知和商品推广语篇提供了一些方法。

　　传统的语法方法更注重语言形式、结构以及对音素、语素、句法等不同层次内部关系的描述或解释，而以认知为基础的语法方法则充分强调认知主体的功能、认知方法和概念系统。语法的认知方法以语言系统为核心。虽然约翰·泰勒（John Taylor）（Taylor 1995）提出认知语义学的研究是在"认知语法"的框架内进行的，但迪尔克·吉拉兹（Dirk Geeraerts）（Geeraerts 2010）和莱纳德·泰尔米（Leonard Talmy）（Talmy 1988）对认知语法的主张更符合罗纳德·兰艾克（Ronald Langacker）的方法（Langacker 1987a，1991）。后者侧重于语言的意义，例如，在认知语法、空间思维中，语言会影响人们对空间关系和方向的思考、记忆和推理。在过去的十多年中，神经生物学在有关感知、评估、注意力和记忆等方面取得了实质性进展。例如，在词汇层面，有学者认为认知可以被合理地理解为包括对词汇刺激的感知、对刺激的情绪评价、对刺激的注意、对记忆的刺激，以及随后在行为中使用相关信息。脑干、脑边缘系统和脑前边缘区域构成了刺激评估系统（Abutalebi & Clahsen 2015）。因此，在大脑中，情绪和认知是可区分但不可分割的。从神经的角度来看，情感是认知的组成部分。

　　在语义层面，兰艾克（Langacker 1987a）指出诸如名词、动词、形容词和副词之类的基本语法类别在语义上是可定义的。他认为任何语言表达都会激活几个认知域，亦称为复杂矩阵（complex matrix）。认知语法通过主要领域来定义典型词的成员。兰艾克将名词定义为一个事或物，名词归属于一个域；动词是在时间域中对过程的描述；而介词、形容词和副词等也被纳入一个时间域中。过程和时间关系的区别在于心智扫描的不同方式。过程是顺序扫描，通过过程扫描我们可以观察场景每个阶段是如何变化和发展的。整个概念化是动态的，其内容总是在变化的。时间关系则是总体扫描，通过时间扫描，我们以累积的方式观察一个场景的各个方面，并逐渐构建成一个复杂的概念。

　　在语篇层面，兰艾克认为认知语法的方法主要集中在语篇构建和理解的认知加工方面。一方面，认知语法聚焦于语言表达和话语解释；另一方面，认知语法侧重于影响读者的背景知识以及他们如何解读某一特定表达中物质的、社会的和语言内容的能力（Langacker 2008）。换句话说，认知语法致力于探索文本是如何形成、接收和评估的。在语篇研究中，认知语法的基础应用主要探讨了识解在文学语篇中（Harrison et al. 2014；严天欣 2021）以及其他语篇中的作用（Hart 2014；Zhang & Luo 2017）。与词项一样，话语的意义由概念内容和特定的内容识解组成。例如，有学者发现，认知识解是在文学作品中创造意义的语言工具（Stockwell 2009）。严天欣（2021）从认知识解的角度分析了小说《使女的故事》的语法特征。其研究发现，"扫描过滤"和"详略度选择"等策略有助于从心理和意识形态角度诠释对小说主题的不同理解。哈特（Hart 2014）在媒体话语中描述了功能语法、多模态语法和认知语法作为语言模型在揭示社会和政治语境中话语的意识形态特征方面的作用。哈特的主要论点是，理解语言所必然涉及的认知过程是基于视觉体验的。一些西方学者将认知语法扩展到语篇研究层面，在分析当代小说时采用动作链、参考点模式、剖析和构图路径等理论（比如 Harrison et al. 2014）；在我国，张辉和罗一丽（2017）通过认知语法的视角对战略情报话语进行了批判性认知分析，以扩展其在情报分析中的作用。以上所有尝试都证实了认知语法理论在话语研究中应用的有效性。

目前，认知语言学学者从不同的角度对认知语法进行了相关研究。这一领域的研究与句法、词法、认知语言学、认知语法构建中的语法学等其他领域相结合，取得了许多成果。一些学者甚至设法将这一理论应用于语言教学和语言习得。显然，更多关于认知语法的内容需要进一步开发。认知语法可能在语言学习中起到促进作用。此外，很少有研究从社会语言学和实证研究的角度对认知语法进行分析。笔者将认知语法与语篇相结合进行的研究尝试对认知构建和语篇意义释解进行系统的探究，相信随着研究的不断深入，人们对认知语法的认识会不断更新。

本书以医疗产品和服务推广语篇为研究对象，以认知语法为研究视角，探讨跨文化认知构建差异及认知差异导致的不同的语用策略。本书进行的是跨学科和跨领域的复合研究，此研究模式也是当前"新文科"研究的新趋势，即以实证研究为手段，探讨"商务+医学+认知+语言"的内涵和实践运用，以及跨文化认知语言在特定医疗推广语境中的语用差异，在认知语言学理论发展、商务推广语篇分析和应用语言学研究领域都具有一定的创新意义。

其一，跨文化探讨商务医疗语篇中语言生成、识解、认知构建与医学、商务、社会、机构、群体和个人交流的关联，可以提升跨文化认知能力，并为语言实证研究和社会语言学研究提供新的研究思路，为规范医疗语篇和产品促销语篇提供交际实践借鉴。

其二，跨文化综合分析人文和科学动态发展和横向交叉发展情况以及它们对现实语境沟通的影响，强调新语境下医学和商务沟通语篇中的认知模式，可以在语言学理论建设和产品推广方面提供文化的、系统的和具有特色的跨学科研究基础。

其三，通过跨文化实证方式分析认知模式和语言选择的语法结构和语言表达差异，丰富社会语言学、跨文化交际的研究内容和范畴。

其四，跨文化探索医疗推广语篇中的社会、医学和语言因素，科学分析医疗语篇所体现的认知语言机制和医疗推广语篇的话语促进手段，为当今中国产品国际化提供语言理论指导、语言建制以及跨文化人工智能交际复制的研究基础。

通过对企业产品推广语篇的实证分析，笔者认为，在多文化语境中必定存在多层次的多样认知。通过对不同文化语境中某个特定商业群体的语用行为进行定性和定量分析我们可以了解他们多样性的认知，而这些多样性认知是如何影响商品的市场推广结果的？本书通过语言识解来解读认知语法和词汇选择，研究具有不同文化背景、有着不同认知经验的交际者进行了什么样的涉及认知语言学的语法选择（例如情态动词或名词短语）和意义识解，以及对商业和市场推广产生了哪些不同的影响。正如一些学者所提出的，在交际中，简单的语言区分抑或选择会造成交际的冲突或资源再分配的缺失（Desmet et al. 2016）。跨文化共同认知可以促进商业交际和产品的推广，不同的语言认知可能会对产品推广产生障碍。例如：产品进入他文化市场的过程是具有不同文化背景的群体在语言识解过程中进行协调和沟通的过程。

由于企业在开展国际业务时可能会面对经济、技术和文化等方面的各种变化，企业话语语篇作者应通过参与跨文化认知活动来适应新的文化环境，如加强对全球化、科学技术进步和企业日益增加的社会责任的认知可以帮助不同文化背景的语篇作者了解如何构建适合他文化背景下的市场和消费群体。此外，商业环境的快速变化，加上企业受利润驱动需要不断占领市场并拓展新客户或留住老客户，这些都促使语篇作者意识到语言语用的重要性：语篇中的语言语用不仅是为了构建自我意识，也是为了构建对来自其他文化的读者或潜在客户的认知。因此，对真实企业推广语篇语言及其数据的分析就非常重要，特别是对当代企业中大量对内、对外沟通话语和语篇的研究，这些话语语篇不仅体现了企业的沟通技术、流派、风格、目标，而且可以洞察语篇中的语言语用在沟通中的协同作用和功能，这些无疑可以帮助我们解读语篇背后的认知构建，并预测语篇可能导致阅读群体的认知（差异）。因此，跨文化认知话语研究有助于考察企业如何通过语言与员工和利益相关者进行互动，与目标市场、现有客户和整个世界进行互动，以及这些企业的整体公众形象是如何在内部和外部构建的。

从书中的实证分析结果来看，笔者认为企业期望通过话语语篇构建的认知包含两种相互关联的方式。一个是对企业宣传意图、营销目标、企业身份的认知过程，该过程是通过一系列嵌入企业文化和价值观的机构话语语篇来维持的。另一个是公司针对他文化目标读者（如投资者、客户和公众）在语篇中的语言语用，也就是企业自我概念的语篇实践表达。这两个关联方式共同帮助企业在他文化语境构建积极或负面的企业形象，并为其商业宣传行为提供合法性。因此，企业推广话语语篇，作为一种包含功利价值观和商业目标的亚里士多德语言表征，应该在社会成员之间创造一种共同感和共同认知，即商业话语针对的不仅是内部读者，而且也包含外部读者，他们在不同文化背景下都会接受并支持该公司的商业行动，比如产品推销。公司的商业信誉以及企业精神，是通过跨文化认知意识和恰当的语言应用、沟通策略、话语中的意识形态机制等共同构建的。此语篇中的组合构建是语篇作者专门设计语用策略，以实现提升企业声誉（比如通过使用"成熟的/稳定的"或"公认的/认可的"等表述来构建大众认知）和自我推销（比如通过形象展示和身份宣传来构建对企业的认知）的目的，从而使多种认知组合更具有持久性，助力公司向具有不同文化背景的、不同专业水平的乃至全世界的目标读者提供有效的正面宣传。

总之，认知是一个非常复杂的内外兼顾的内化过程，这一过程体现了一个个性化、自然化、民族化和知识化构建的复杂体系和庞大工程。从有限的外在经验推导出无限的知识构建，个人自我的有限认知如何能和知识相结合运用于具体交际实践，比如个人的语言认知如何体现在对外推广语篇中，仍然存在很大的研究空间。话语语篇策略显现认知过程，涉及语言结构中的语篇构架、句法、词项和语法及其文化的隐性解读，对其中的认知探索和逻辑构建仍然是应用语言学很热门的一个研究领域，但如何在跨文化语境中对认知语篇进行实证研究，仍需要进一步探索，比如是否需要考虑对语篇作者进行访谈以增加分析的可信度。认知语言学所涉及的语言表征既有逻辑性也有文化性，它在具体交际语篇中才可以被真切地感知和认识，从而转化为有意义的语言交际。

本书是作者在医疗商务语境下对认知语言学进行的实证研究。文皓竣、王一然、肖美儿为本书第四、第五和第六章研究数据的整理和分析做了一些工作；此外，本书在语言修正方面还得到了丁洋岚、贺宇萌、李欣叶、李之松、马晓楠等同学的帮助，在此表示衷心感谢。本书的出版得到了广东外语外贸大学外国语言学及应用语言学研究中心、广东外语外贸大学高等教育"冲补强"专项资金项目以及广东松山职业技术学院（笔者是该学院的首聘北江讲座教授）的课题赞助，同时科学出版社的编辑对本书的出版也给予了大力的支持和指导，在此一并感谢。认知语言学的研究方兴未艾，在分析中由于涉及跨文化个人体验和认知能力差异，以及文化、政治和教育背景等影响个人体验和认知能力的因素繁多，笔者主要是基于文本语言和语法表征进行解读，很难在动态发展的社会的、文化的、政治的和个人特性的方面进行更为细致的分析和解读，疏漏之处在所难免。笔者希望此书能抛砖引玉，也期望越来越多具有批判性的、更科学的、多角度的、多层面的研究问世，使应用语言学、认知语言学、商务语篇分析和特殊用途英语（语言）的研究有可持续性的长足发展。

杨文慧

2023 年 11 月

Contents

Abbreviations

Ago	Agonist
Ago+/Agonist+	stronger Agonist
AI	artifical intelligence
AML	Acute Myeloid Leukemia
Ant	Antagonist
Ant+/Antagonist+	stronger Antagonist
AUX	auxiliary
BRI	Belt and Road Initiative
BS	basic space
C	Conceptualizer
CA	conversation analysis
CAQCS	computer assisting quantitative cumulative system
CBT	Cognitive Blending Theory
CDA	critical discourse analysis
CG	cognitive grammar
CIF	cost, insurance and freight
CL	cognitive linguistics
CT	Chinese text
DAPT	Dual Anti-Platelet Therapy
DI	default inheritance
DST	Discourse Space Theory
EB	establishing backgrounds
EC	establishing credentials
ECM	Event-domain Cognitive Model

ES	event space
ESL	English as a Second Language
ESP	English for Specific Purposes
ET	English text
HIV	human immunodeficiency virus
ICM	idealized cognitive model
IO	introducing the offer
IS	immediate scope
M	Move
MDPNs	medical device promotion news
MOOCs	Massive Open Online Courses
MS	maximal scope
NLP	natural language process
O	object of conception
OI	offering incentives
PMDA	Pharmaceuticals and Medical Devices Agency
PoV	point of view
R&D	research and development
S	subject of conception
SaaS	software as a service
SFL	Systematic functional linguistics
TCT	Thinprep Cytologic Test
TM	Trend Micro
Tr	trajector
V	viewer
VF	viewing frame
WG	word grammar

Chapter 1

Introduction to Media Promotional Discourse Studies

As members of any society, individuals' understanding of the world relies on their unique beliefs, values, and cultures, which vary across countries, ethnic groups, regions, and communities. In this regard, cognitive differences ubiquitously exist in China and other countries as well in aspects of history, cultural customs, language habits, social systems. The centred attention on cognitive linguistics (CL) in this book rests on its core epistemological idea of experientialism and linguistic behaviour, highlighting the bodily and spatial experience in the course of human social activities under a specific cultural setting (the promoting setting of medical products and service), which provides fruitful anchor points for the combination of cognitive linguistics and cross-cultural studies for business communication, delving into their relationships with underlying values, thinking patterns, and ideologies in societies. Linguistic studies, on the one hand, require cross-cultural comparisons to establish connections between linguistic phenomena and cultural issues, thereby enhancing their practical relevance for institutions and individuals in commercial contexts. On the other hand, the limited analysis of language use represents a significant shortcoming in cross-cultural studies, considering that language constitutes an indispensable component of cognitive science and culture. While considerable efforts have been dedicated to cognitive linguistics at the lexical or semantic level, this book aims to exploit and refine a more comprehensive methodology or perspective. This endeavour calls for the creative integration of both semantic and discoursal theoretical viewpoints within authentic professional texts.

1.1   Research Background

Evidently, as cognitive science expands the notion of motivation to include its cognitive impact on psychology and sociology, it also acknowledges the importance of various domains of linguistic description, such as pragmatics and discourse studies. The study of cognitive linguistics in a cross-cultural context, particularly in the Sino-American medical fields, is motivated by several factors. First, both the United States and China hold significant economic positions in the world. Second, the United States dominates the medical field, while China experiences rapid medical development. Third, the global health landscape has been reshaped in the wake of the recent pandemic.

Regarding economic development, China has gained rapid growth. China's Belt and Road Initiative (BRI), since its inception, has sparked extensive discussions domestically and internationally, eliciting diverse interpretations. The successful implementation of this initiative depends not only on the cooperation of countries directly involved in the BRI project but also on the participation of developed nations, particularly the United States. Given its significant roles in political, military, and economic realms worldwide, the United States aims to assert its influence by restricting the execution of China's BRI project. However, it is worth noting that the "New Silk Road" announced by former Secretary of State Hillary Rodham Clinton in 2011 overlaps with China's BRI, necessitating further discussion and cooperation between China and the United States in the shared regions. This complex relationship, involving world trade and political interests, has become a key issue in balancing the global economy, requiring careful consideration by both nations. Any proposed changes by China or the United States will have significant impacts on the countries involved. Especially in the aftermath of the 2020 pandemic, the promotion of professional health-related products is of paramount importance in many countries. This highlights the essential role played by the Chinese people in the process of economic evolution and development. The customers' perception of professional products not only shapes institutional strategies but also influences the direction and extent of scientific development and national investment in healthcare fields.

Meanwhile, as the growing health concern among the public requires leading medical products and treatment, the global medical production and service market is expanding. Global health and its marketization gradually force medical companies to be internationalized. Market penetration and revenue generation propel these companies to be ever more competitive. This case is more serious in markets of medicine and medical treatment which are now dominated by advanced North American and European companies under the circumstances of the pandemic and severe illness, while only limited medical companies and institutions in China have gained worldwide recognition. With its economic development, China's medical companies also manage to earn their places and build positive reputations in the medical market, and their published discourses are considered as important sources for promoting products, beliefs and companies themselves. Therefore, the significance of language use in promotional discourses speaks for companies. As it is well documented that East Asians differ from Westerners in conscious perception and attention (Nisbett & Miyamoto 2005), this book will examine the cognitive mechanism embedded in language use in both English and Chinese promotional discourses to identify the cross-cultural cognitive differences in promoting languages, giving insights on cognition construction in the West and East to improve the mutual understanding and international marketization of the products.

People across the world pay great attention to the development of medical products, medical devices, treatment, and government policies in China. The manufacture of medicines and development of treatments are always what people concern the most whenever they run into pandemics or other diseases, along with their mass production and promotion. To share the international markets, medical companies, research institutions and pharmaceutical factories attract attention from investors, journalists, shareholders, and potential buyers by publishing news, advertisements and press releases related to new medicines, medical devices and treatment on their own websites to disseminate product information, maintain visibility and acquire readers and possible users. Yet, the types of medicines, devices and treatment, along with their R&D (research and development) processes and ways of application, varied from each other and different brands, bringing about different understandings and interpretations to users and consumers. Taking the two leading countries in vaccine manufacturing for instance, China and the U.S., Chinese pharmaceutical companies such as Sinopharm and Sinovac develop their vaccines based on inactivated viruses while those from America, such as Johnson & Johnson and Pfizer, mainly produce viral vector vaccines or encapsulated mRNA vaccines. It may be difficult for consumers or vaccine receivers to figure out the differences between the vaccines produced in China and the U.S., so as to make a decision for purchase from the two. Although the governments in different nations will mandatorily require their citizens to get vaccinated, while some of them choose to receive vaccines produced by their own country, others might choose those manufactured in other countries. For those relatively small countries that are not capable of producing vaccines themselves, they need to make choices on purchasing and importing vaccines from other countries. Then how Chinese pharmaceutical companies promote their medical products to other countries and meet international standards touches on essential cognitive issues regarding intercultural communication in medical fields.

Cognitive study furnishes a paradigm that considers the relationship between language and our perception and conceptualization. As a branch of cognitive science, cognitive linguistics views language as part of the human cognitive system which comprises different cognitive abilities (Dirven & Verspoor 2004). That is, language correlates to human minds, and, to a great extent, reflects human thinking patterns and language behaviour. Language delivers ideas, opinions or ideologies, and discourses, as the carrier of language, are embodied with human cognition, demonstrating attitudes, beliefs and values toward the world. Grounded on the above assumptions, cognitive linguists constantly devote themselves to the study of relationships between human cognitive abilities and grammatical constructions or language uses (Langacker 1999).

Recently, the research of cognitive linguistics on commercial discourses mainly focuses on lexical devices, such as metaphor usages in commodity distribution and promotional discourses (e.g. Caballero 2009; Yang 2020), image schema in sports business discourses (e.g. Yang 2020), and roles in achieving the persuasive purpose (e.g. Bhatia 2005; Breeze 2013; Jaworska

2017), which leaves gaps on studies of syntax, grammar and discoursal perspectives which also construct the meanings in texts and represent cognitive positions at the same time. Croft and Cruse (2004: 247) initiate that a construction as a unit cuts across the componential model of grammatical knowledge. According to them, constructions, like the lexical items in the lexicon, are "vertical" structure that combines syntactic, semantic and even phonological information. At grammatical levels, Bybee (1985) presents the evidence that semantic similarity of grammatical units, such as words, plays an important role in the organization of grammatical knowledge in a speaker's mind. Thus, Croft and Cruse (2004: 307) propose four hypotheses about the effects of language use on grammatical representation. The first one is the independent representation of an infected word form as a function of its token frequency in language use. The second is the productivity of rule/schema as a function of a high type frequency of low token frequency instances, not of the structural openness of the schema. The third is that schemas can be formed from members of an inflectional category from a source form. Lastly, the organization of inflected word forms is influenced by the degree of semantic similarity between word forms. However, there is less authentic evidence to support these hypotheses at activation levels of entrenched constructions whose structure might not match authentic utterances or texts in cross-cultural contexts, as Croft (1998) argues that it is possible that speakers might not have the most schematic construction represented in their minds if they are not activated sufficiently.

In this book, the author cross-culturally examines grammatical representations of words, what they represent and the processes they are involved in within both English and Chinese discourses, in the hope of identifying the type and token frequency that plays distinct roles in the empirical analyses of grammar-based patterns for cognition construction. Authentic and concrete supporting evidence from the empirical and contrastive studies will be put forward on the nature of grammar construction, including the role of token frequency in metonymic applications associated with PoV, the role of type frequency of verb stimuli in discourses associated with force dynamics productivity, the formation of modalities in entrenchments and groundings within sentences, and their emergencies of generalizations in medical discoursal interpretations. By doing the series of cognitive grammar studies in medical promotional discourses, it is possible to identify different kinds of cognitive operations, processes and models on which they can work by interpreting the uses of language in both English and Chinese commercial contexts. This is the first goal of this book. Another goal is to provide linguistic evidence that cognitive operations relating to cognitive grammar (CG) can underlie the interpretations of utterances in different grammar repositories as well as at different levels of meaning construction. To this end, the author chooses the word grammar and its related repositories, a usage-based account of language-based meaning construction that reconciles insights from cognitive-oriented constructionist perspectives (cf. Ruiz de Mendoza & Mairal 2008, 2011).

1.2   Institutional Discourses

Institutional discourse analysts do not consider language in isolation as their object of study, but they seek to establish how written discourses and spoken texts reflect the social and organizational contexts in which they are used for business and operation purposes. As Bourdieu (1991) sees it, an institution doesn't refer to a certain or a particular organization, but is a relatively stable combination of social relations that endows individuals with power, status and resources of various sorts. An institution has its own sets of independent value systems, and makes judgments about what is right or wrong and deals with them technically in accordance with national laws and regulations as well as relevant government rules. In addition, institutions determine their own work contents and service recipients based on their roles in social operation (Wodak 1996). So we can see that institutions play important roles in the process of constructing social orders and making them parts of the common sense of the public. To communicate with the public, institutions develop their own ways to form their characteristics and uniqueness in operation, production and management. Language, as a typical construction of institutional characteristics and uniqueness, is the means of communication, through which individuals or institutions can express themselves and convey information to the internal staff and external public. Deetz (1982) claims that language is one of the fundamental elements in constituting the operation mechanism of various organizations and institutions. Andrea (2004) also proposes that language works as the major means of constructing social reality and identity for different kinds of organizations and institutions. Similarly, Li (2016) argues that there is no prior or objective reason for the existence of a particular institution, including its entity, mission, function and value systems. Rather, all of these need to be demonstrated by a series of descriptions, illustrations and argumentation, i.e. the selection of discourse resources and lexis, and then the existence of an institution can be endowed with legality by the society. Thus, based on the views about the relationship between language and institutions, in this sense, the illocutionary act of institutions and the fact that institutions construct their identities through discourses make it a significant attempt to probe into the deep meaning of the superficial language use and linguistic features of discourses issued by different sorts of institutions.

Initially, institutional discourse is a kind of social act or interaction within the particular cultural context of a society. When regarded as a social act, discourse implicates a particular purpose and may lead to a certain outcome (Miao 2006). Schiffrin et al. (2001) point out that discourse is the interaction and communication between members of a society and it's also the social practice in which members of the society employ language resources to fulfil various tasks in social life. In a word, there is a close association between discourse and society, and discourse plays an important part in various areas of social life. That is also one of the reasons that social issues have always been the key point of discourse analysis. However, relevant research is presented in these areas, including critical discourse analysis (CDA), institutional discourse analysis, political discourse analysis, media discourse analysis and so on (Miao 2006), among which institutional discourse has attracted the eyeballs of many researchers in recent years because it is related to authentic communication in various professions and institutions, usually occurring in a particular business setting or interaction, often affected by sets of institutional rules and professional principles with specific purposes (Guo 2015), such as company promotional discourses, advertising discourses, legislative discourses, court trials, news interviews, doctor-patient interactions, classroom communication, political discourses. Institutional discourses like company websites, reviews, and sponsorships are both vertical and horizontal interactivities (such as the interaction of design and information). As suggested by Breeze (2013: 152), people explore websites by traversing hyperlinks from one webpage to another, their ability to build a model in their mind of what the website has to tell them is influenced by the interplay between the site's content organization, its design and its navigability features.

1.2.1 The research scope of institutional discourses

Institutional discourse analysis examines how people use language to accomplish a task or activity and reach the set goal in public institutional contexts such as teaching, medicine, counselling, interrogation, negotiation and interviews (Miao 2006). Discourse practice is the way and media for institutions to fulfil their social duties, convey information about their products or services and express themselves. Based on the classification of discourse which is communicative discourse and strategic discourse, Habermas (1984) regards institutional discourse as a strategic discourse, which presents a specific purpose of the agent and differences in power status, involving the process of the exchange of information between the institution and the contexts. From the view of Levinson (1992), institutional discourse is goal-oriented or task-oriented, containing various constraints on the achievement of goals or tasks as well as particular forms of reasoning by participants when they decode and interpret the discourse. Drew and Heritage (1992) consider institutional discourse as a variation and deviation from the communicative system of language and they have summed up three characteristics of it: (i) institutional discourse is carried out with a specific goal; (ii) the participation of different parts of interlocutors in the interaction of discourse is constrained to varying degrees; (iii) there is a corresponding framework of reasoning for a particular institutional context. In addition, scholars, by examining public institutional discourses, mainly focus on the asymmetry of rights, and how interlocutors play different roles to influence the discourse structure and its development trajectory (Holmes & Stubbe 2003; Mayr 2004). In this branch, Thornborrow (2002) proposes four characteristics of public institutional discourses when they are viewed as means of interactions: (i) interlocutors have distinguished roles that are pre-marked; (ii) the asymmetry of turns; (iii) the asymmetry of rights and obligations of the interlocutors; and (iv) the discourse resources and the role of the interlocutors are strengthened or weakened in a particular institutional context. These characteristics also provide insights for other types of institutional discourse analysis.

Lü and Huang (2015) further point out that the task-oriented nature of professional activities and the pre-marking of the interlocutors' institutional identities are the necessary elements, i.e. the primary elements in constituting the institutional discourse. The asymmetry of discourse power, the constraint of professional activity procedures, the strategy of discourse selection and the specificity of discourse reasoning are the secondary characteristics of institutional discourse, which are derived from the primary elements. Among multiple factors that influence communication, identity and power are two major factors that are non-negligible in institutional discourse analysis. To demonstrate the appropriateness of the principle of goal direction, a new approach to pragmatics in institutional discourse analysis, Lü and Huang (2015) also illustrate the relationship between the communicative goal, identity and power in the contexts of institutional discourse, which are helpful for us to understand the nature of institutional discourse and to do analysis. Simply speaking, that is: interlocutors with different identities have their own communicative goals, which might be consistent, conflicting or neutral, thus forming the specific relationship of goals among interlocutors. On the other hand, different identities endow discourse interlocutors with specific power, and then interlocutors can achieve their communicative goals through discourses that are in line with their identities (i.e. role-playing). During the communication, power differences can exert a force that restrains the achievement of goals. These abstract notions are ultimately realized and constructed through language use and details in interactions (Lü & Huang 2015). Therefore, the communicative goals of the institution, the identity and power of different parts of interlocutors, as well as the relationship and force formed in the discourse need to be considered in institutional discourse contexts.

Institutional discourse and its research scope in fact employ all of the research approaches to reveal how companies communicate with different audiences—employees, customers, investors, communities, and societies—through lexical, written, verbal, visual, generic, and other specific features. The research results provide a comprehensive overview of how companies communicate, what they communicate, and what effects of the communication, aiming to "identify discourse strategies, document trends and developments, and illuminate the ongoing relationships that companies build with a variety of stakeholders in today's increasingly complex business environment" (Breeze 2013: 1). Its research scope consists of broad perspectives not only on the various discursive practices as social acts of business, but also on the various methodological ways by which the analysts conduct the research, illustrating either straightforward or theoretical ways how institutional discourse writers construct their institutional, professional and social roles through their discourses. As Breeze (2013: 23) argues, corporate/constitutional discourse is "the total communication activities of a company at various levels", and institutional discourse should be understood as a discourse system consisting of a set of discourses divided into (1) speakers or "origins" (discourses generated by the company) and (2) assumed "receivers" (e.g. employees, customers, investors, and the general public); (3) the major forms or "genres" of textual expression (e.g. employee handbooks, promotional magazines, annual reports) and (4) "discourse types" or categories (e.g. promotional, informational, legitimating discourses). Each of these discourses places the company within and outside the institutional world, and elaborates on the importance of institutional discourse in the ongoing shaping of society.

Generally, three different groups of researchers study institutional discourses with different research methods and hold different opinions. Professional groups and English teaching specialists tend to have a specific and practical focus, while applied linguists and discourse analysts may often be more theoretical (Breeze 2013). The professional groups conduct studies by taking the company's benefits (i.e. enlarging market share, uplifting corporate reputation, etc.) as the starting point. Applied linguists and discourse analysts usually study discourses neutrally and critically, as they are not bound by any company and their main focus is on how language works in sociological or philosophical contexts. English teaching specialists aim to make business language knowledge accessible to non-native English users. Although these three different groups use different theories, and have different findings, yet their approaches to carrying out the research often overlap. In addition to the above, Breeze uses a different textual (i.e. corpus, genre and multimodal) approach to corporate/institutional discourses, as well as the social (i.e. ethnographic and intercultural) ones. Such a corpus approach is often used in a qualitative way to deal with a collection of texts, and a representative of particular genres, which usually provides a greater degree of objectivity. Under the multimodal approaches, language is not the only way that the entities want to communicate with the world. For instance, advertising, corporate websites or online newspapers containing moving images, sound, and videos are all multimodal. This approach is considered as a critical approach, or CDA not as a method, but as an attitude or a way of thinking about texts. In recent years, institutional discourse in fact includes many different approaches including corpus analysis, systemic functional linguistics, qualitative text analysis, ethnography, multimodal studies, even conversation analysis (CA, a conventional method which has derived from ethnomethodology). For the social approaches, on the one hand, ethnographic approaches develop an insider's view qualitatively, usually through observation or interviews. The rich descriptions of situations and contexts they provide can help researchers and business practitioners to understand and draw conclusions beyond immediate context and shed light on the nature of the wider social contexts. On the other hand, many intercultural approaches aim to describe and interpret cultural variations through the lens of socio-anthropology and cultural theories, which help to unveil culture-salient corporate discourse (Jiang 2014). Nevertheless, examining institutional discourse, both internal and external, not only benefits society and individuals, but also advances our research and pedagogy in professional communication (Bhatia 2004).

1.2.2　Studies of institutional media discourses

With the rapid development of globalization and the change of marketization, the way institutions establish identities, construct reality and make speech events by employing discourses changed a lot. Remarkable achievements have been made in discourses issued by institutions on their products or services from various perspectives (Harvey 2013; Izquierdo & Blanco 2020; Kaur et al. 2013; Xiong 2012; Xiong & Li 2020). Many studies by Fairclough (1992) have revealed the effect of the expansion of the market economy on Western institutional discourses. It is found that, advertisements, counselling activities and market economy have an influence on the context of institutional discourse in the time of marketization, leading to the trend of technicalization and marketization of institutional discourse, which covers the traditional format and styles of discourse and obscures the original power relationship (Li 2016). Apart from move structures or generic patterns identified at the discoursal level, what is believed to be important is the communicative purposes researchers have explored. Language in promotional discourses issued on institutional websites is both informational and promotional (Bhatia 2005). Presenting a full picture of a company and its product or service is the fundamental role of institutional discourses. And there does exist much research on their institutional function. For instance, Xiong's (2012) genre analysis of universities' academic job advertisements in newspapers, shows that rhetorical moves and discursive strategies are employed for self-advertising such as branding universities as well as informing the academic posts. Xiong and Li (2020), based on their corpus-based analysis of the marketization of higher education on the universities' official websites, add new evidence in support of self-advertising as if institutions were business agents competing to sell their products and services to consumers. Additionally, Harvey (2013) conducts a critical multimodal analysis of commercial loss put forward by institutions and reveals that institutional discourses make a huge difference to consumers' perception of products by either transforming ailments into severe ones or confusing them as a treatable illness. Izquierdo and Blanco (2020), by conducting English-Spanish contrastive analyses, further find that in herbal tea texts issued by pharmaceutical producers, discursive strategies like emotion-laden strategies and reason-based strategies are widely adopted respectively for product sales.

Except for the features of the product itself, some cultural or social ideologies are embedded in an institutional discourse which reshapes readers' consumption view and convinces them to believe the values of the product (Kaur et al. 2013). For instance, under the background of the increasing prices of real estate that severely affect the national economy and citizens' lives, Li (2016) analyses the advertisements of real-estate developers, revealing how commercial institutions promote their values to the society by using discourses and how these discourses exert impacts on the ideologies and relationship in Chinese societies. Chen (2016) examines the advertisements produced by four top-selling automobile brands in China. By focusing on the multimodal discursive means through which the concept of "nature" is constructed, the research reveals a consistent ideological separation between nature and human society in the analyzed advertisements, contributing to the studies on green marketing discourses. Besides, adopting a corpus-driven critical discourse analysis approach, Misir and Işik-Güler (2022) investigate the promotional materials of the online learning platforms Massive Open Online Courses (known as MOOCs). Their findings show that MOOC platforms' marketing language promotes an ideal subject that fits in a neoliberal job market and figures out an array of promotional persuasion strategies of the institution which reinforce a self-betterment discourse to create marketable employees. All in all, institutional discourses not only provide a great amount of information, but also serve the functions of self-advertising and products or services informing, aiming at inducing consumers to believe in what institutions want to deliver.

1.3　Studies of Promotional Discourses

Discourse analysis approach of the promotional discourse revolves around the corpus-based discourse analysis, critical discourse analysis, discourse strategy and so on by focusing on topics ranging from industry sales to public policies. Promotional discourses exhibit a purposive characteristic, which, as a subdivision of English for Specific Purposes (ESP), is connected with descriptive text types whose goal is to persuade (Biber & Zhang 2018). That is to say, promotional genre is a kind of persuasion together with description, to inform the customers about a given product (Bhatia 2008). Bhatia (2005) claims that the most traditional promotional discourse is what has been known as advertisement, which is often regarded as a system of discourse that contains informative and promotional purposes to persuade chosen people to buy certain ideas, goods and services. Other scholars also associate the connotation of promotional discourses with advertising. Izquierdo and Blanco (2020) argue that promotion is bound up with a broad concept of advertising, which is an activity intended to help to sell a product.

Promotional discourse is tightly associated with business communication, a purposeful social activity that serves to demonstrate an intent or a target which expresses a given community's way of making things happen through language (Swales 2004). Except for linguistics, other disciplines like communication science, psychology and social science all conduct research on discourse analysis. Scholars apply discourse analysis method to investigate texts at various linguistic levels (Miao 2006), such as syntax, semantics, stylistics, etc. Discourse and cognition are inseparable. The communicator's cognition involves not only individual cognition, but also social culture cognition. For one thing, discourse or text is an effective and significant approach to exploring cognition (Virtanen 2004). For another, cognition is an important component of discourse analysis (Semino & Culpeper 2002). Except for cognition, discourse also has a strong correlation with society. Schiffrin et al. (2001) point out that discourses are not only the interactions between social members, but also the social practices that social members use language resources to realize various tasks in social life. As social linguists, Wardhaugh and Fuller (2015) introduce three major approaches to discourse analysis: conversation analysis, international sociolinguistics and CDA, which is designed to discuss the relationship between discourse and social structure from a critical perspective.

Within the last two decades, many analysts of discourse studies for business purposes put great efforts on CDA, and promoting discourse is one of the core interests. Erjavec (2004) adheres to the analytic paradigm of CDA described by Fairclough (1992, 1995), proposing an amalgamated method of text analysis and discourse process analysis to consider the generation and connotation of discourses, combining with the thoughts of ethnography. Erjavec (2004) attempts to prove that this expanded approach is useful and checks it in a study of illegal promotional news discourse. The intention of promotional news discourse is to influence consumers in order to earn profits, through a news form. Fairclough (1992, 1995) suggests that the media discourse analysis should be multidimensional, which means texts must be related to the discourse practice and the social practice of which they are part. Concerning that, Erjavec (2004) discusses three disparate but closely connected dimensions of this communicative event: text, discourse practice and social practice. Critical discourse study of promotional discourses illustrates an attitude, an attempt to provide a different perspective on traditional ways of seeing the world and engaging with it, involving a variety of ideas and motivations for business promotion. As for researchers, it is perhaps possible for them to embrace a reflexive and self-reflexive stance on the subject of the CDA study, the way they study it and in their roles as researchers.

Except for CDA, discourse analysis in promotional discourses has also achieved other results. One of them is the research on identifying promotional strategies. Sulaiman (2014) analyses the textual stylistic features of translated tourism promotional texts for getting extra-textual knowledge to propose effective translation strategies and to find out the stylistic differences and cultural challenges involved. He finds that to translate touristic or any other promotional texts, using the "right" form to persuade consumers is more likely to succeed. Equally important, translating tourism promotional texts without taking up a culturally applicable style is not sufficient for the success of touristic texts. Except for strategies employed in tourism promotional texts, Ruffolo (2015) also reveals some interesting linguistic strategies applied in them. Using the approach of corpus linguistics, he studies the discourses released by hotels that aim to promote their green practices for expressing environmental concerns, and targets to unveil any discursive and linguistic strategy used by the discourse producers, attempting to throw light on the embedded cultural assumptions. In addition to business promotional text studies, self-promotion discourse analyses also have been conducted, such as the academic investigation in rhetoric, composition and applied linguistics (Afros & Schryer 2009). Hyland (2000) describes a variety of rhetorical and linguistic resources the scholars deployed to spotlight the noteworthiness, novelty, and uniqueness of their work. Harwood (2005) also examines the lexicogrammatical signals and first-person pronouns of self-promotion strategy in academic discourses.

Apart from probing into the linguistic strategies adopted in promotional discourses, scholars also bend their efforts to other research interests for conducting discourse analysis. On semantic level, metaphor is one of the most often discussed topics in promotional discourses. Breeze (2013) suggests that metaphoricity and analogy are the most significant qualities of advertisement and make advertisement effective and influential. Jaworska (2017) adopts a corpus-assisted approach to the identification and analysis of metaphors supported by Wmatrix, which commits to delving into the relationship between "distance" and metaphors used in promotional tourism discourses. His study is an attempt to prove whether the promotional tourism discourses with certain destinations, which are culturally and geographically faraway from "home", employ more metaphors than that closer to "home", and how the discourse producers employ conceptual mappings and metaphorical expressions. Abuczki (2009) categorizes metaphors used in advertisements published in one of the most popular women's fashion magazines *Cosmopolitan* in Hungarian, and identifies the corresponding conceptual mappings. Caballero (2009) examines metaphors appearing in wine promotional genres and reveals certain conceptual metaphors like "wine is a living organism", "wine is a textile", and "wine is a building". Regarding other research interests, Cheung (2011) adopts Halliday's (1994) model to conduct a thematic analysis of sales promotion letters to discuss the relationship between theme and transitivity, and expounds on the system's versatility in analysing professional communication texts. Suau-Jiménez (2020) construes the credibility in promotional discourses and commits to explain it through closeness and distance that is revealed by agentive authorial voice.

1.4   Studies of Medical Discourses

With the rapid development of civil policies, management and institutions of medical industry, more scholars have done researches on it, covering a number of areas, such as treatment, medicine and big data. As a branch of ESP, medical discourse is a type of discourse in and about healing, curing, or therapy, expressions of suffering, and relevant language ideologies (Wilce 2009: 199). In recent studies, medical discourses can be roughly divided into two types, verbal and textual.

Conversation analysis is one of the branches of discourse analysis, it is devoted to investigating the interactive processes of participants. Thus verbally, medical discourse analyses focus on authentic doctor-patient conversations by exploring social problems associated with social linguistic characteristics. At the linguistic levels, numerous analyses on turn, turn-taking, sequential organization, repair, gap, and interruption have been conducted. While Pilnick and Dingwall (2001) concentrate on the persistence of asymmetry in medical interactions, Fioramonte and Vásquez (2018) discuss the multi-party talks in medical encounters, including patient family members. Hou and Zhang (2014) attempt to attain an analysis of extreme case formulations in doctor-patient interactions. Despite the above studies on medical conversation analyses, conflict talks in doctor-patient conversations are other hot research topics. However, analyses on verbal medical discourses involve counselling characteristics of institutional and professional purposes together with commercial business. In the conversations, at least one of the participants is a professional person with medical background, and has obvious institutional identities related to their professions and institutional operations. Such a conversation is not free because it serves as a commercial counselling act. Silverman (1997) carries out a study of the tacit communicative skills in interactions between counsellors and clients (patients or patient family members) on informing HIV (human immunodeficiency virus) and treatments. For instance, pre- and post-HIV tests, counselling for hemophiliacs who have become HIV positive through transfusion of infected blood. While the analytical sections are primarily informed by conversation analysis, the core of the study is a systematic investigation of what seem to be clearly important features of HIV counselling, and how advice is given and received.

Textually, Gunnarsson (2006) presents a constructionist perspective on the emergence and development of medical written discourse, and discusses the dynamic process related to cognition, society, and social activities. Carter and Rowley (2008) analyse how if-conditionals are brought into play in three genres of medical discourse: research articles, conference presentations, and editorials. Gallardo and Ferrari (2010) put their focus on the doctors' health. They have studied the health and professional texts written by doctors, and utilized the framework of appraisal theory of SFL (systematic functional linguistics) to assess doctors' health conditions. Although online consultation is a kind of textual discourse, and the contents and functions of online consultations are basically the same as offline face-to-face consultations, its mode is by typing basically. It is a kind of written communication. Many features of oral conversations, such as interruptions and silence are scanty in online consultations. Studies related to this kind of discourse analysis are rare, and thus the author intends to conduct research on it.

1.5   Rationale for Medical Promotional Discourse Studies

The rationale of this present research can be unfolded as follows. Moynihan et al. (2002: 886) reckon that medicine companies participate in "sponsoring the definition of diseases and promoting them to both prescribers and consumers". Medical device is no exception in the way of promotion to gain commercial benefits as the R&D process is time-consuming and needs enormous investment. Many researchers have dedicated themselves to exploring various ways of medicine, medical device and medical service promotion and their marketization. In literature, medical device promotion relies much on print and broadcast advertisements, brochures, pamphlets, websites, conferences, seminars etc. (Conko 2011). The news pages of companies' official websites become the most effective knowledge-transfer tool, through which manufacturers make themselves more recognizable, sell their values and compete for health care needs. They, on the one hand, present a full account of information about clinical outcomes, authoritative certification, product launches or other happenings. Instead of just circulating knowledge, they, on the other hand, also carry promotional purposes as many linguists have identified by examining their generic features (Bhatia 2004; Erjavec 2004; Maat 2007). However, promotional materials which may contain misleading information with regard to the use of medical devices or their properties are strictly prohibited under government regulations, such as the medical regulations in China. The attractive language is therefore regulated, and it is thus important to explore how these texts operate to influence readers' expectations and decisions.

Traditionally, there are two tendencies in the study of promotional discourses, namely, the tendency of in-depth development and the tendency of horizontal development. The former refers to the in-depth research of linguistics, while the latter refers to the interdisciplinary combination of linguistics and other disciplines to solve various complex language problems through interdisciplinary research on language. Moreover, from the current situation of contemporary linguistic research, this "interdisciplinary tendency" is more obvious. As Shu (2008) suggests, meaning is cantered in cognitive linguistics studies. The encoding and decoding of the meaning in the discourse require the employment of various cognitive mechanisms, such as reasoning, inferring, and conceptualizing. Understanding the meaning of the discourse, therefore, involves more than decoding the surfaced structure and literal meaning; it also involves the identification of the "embodied mind" beneath the discourse. Cognitive Linguistics, formed by the combination of linguistics and cognitive science, is the embodiment of the horizontal development trend of linguistic research, which underlies the human conceptual system and plays a central role in human cognition that is deeply entrenched in recurring patterns of bodily experience and meaning interpretations of language production. Hence, it is essential to study the cognition construction to reveal the true meanings in discourses and interaction communication in order to create mutual understanding across cultures and at the same time to serve international business.

The attempt of writing this book to employ a cognitive grammar approach to English and Chinese promotional discourses in medical device industry is motivated by the following linguistic theoretical and practical marketing considerations. Firstly, from the linguistic perspective, previous studies of cognitive linguistics regarding syntax are said to be at an underdeveloped status. Especially in recent accounts, semantic and syntactic research within the field has been dispositional to be more abstract and conceptual, such as studies on metaphor and metonymy as well as frame semantics and construal. Given this, some scholars propose to do linguistic research based on the combination of cognitive linguistics and Functional Grammar. Yet this new strand has not been practiced in real-life conversations or discourses for specific purposes, i.e. a usage-based application. Moreover, previous research within the field of cognitive linguistics is mainly based on naturally occurring sentences and linguistic data without giving due attention to language used for special purposes or on specific occasions, such as medical promotional discourses. Particularly in such a pandemic situation, the importance of interpreting the medical-related discourse is self-evident. Secondly, it is also necessary to conduct a comparative study on promotional discourses as internationalization becomes an irresistible trend. The conceptualizations that are expressed in natural language have an experiential basis, i.e. they link up with the way in which human beings experience reality, both culturally and physiologically. Therefore, knowledge that is skilfully expressed depends on what values and beliefs people hold. It warns that we have to be sensitive to cultural differences in order to obtain a global view versus a local view. The cross-cultural cognitive differences and similarities revealed in English and Chinese promotional discourses might uncover the hidden ideologies of both Chinese and English writers, hoping to clear cultural and social barriers in promoting medical appliances, such as coronary stents, in the future. Thirdly, the demand for medical devices is increasing as medical treatment now becomes a top priority for people's health and quality of life. Medical device companies compete for sales fiercely. As a result, they constantly disseminate positive clinical and patient-centred outcomes which offer valuable insights for consumers into the possible effects of treatment. News and press releases are promotional materials available on the company's official websites to refer to information about clinical outcomes, authoritative certification, product launches or other happenings. Instead of just circulating knowledge, they also carry promotional purposes as many linguists have identified by examining their generic features (Bhatia 2004; Erjavec 2004; Maat 2007). They advocate positive aspects of products to the extent that their products are of the best quality, the author thinks that it is significant to explore the cognitive process of how discourse producers construct discourses and market their products within.

1.6   The Main Content of the Book

In the book, the author focuses her attention on grammatical evidence for cognitive modelling, i.e. the activity of cognitive operations and processes on cognitive models. Accordingly, this book falls into the category of medical discourse studies and language studies. Language is formed on the basis of interactive experience and cognition process in the real world, which is one of the most explicit ways for human beings to express thoughts, and modern linguistic studies show that cognition and language are inextricably linked. People can consequently believe that cognition is closely related to our consciousness and thinking patterns because language is deeply rooted in human cognitive structure. The book contains seven chapters. Chapter 1 lays down the research background and rationale of medical promotional discourse studies. In Chapter 2, the author offers theoretical considerations and research frame for the present study, and it tackles the issue of adequacy in cognitive linguistic studies and presents the cognitive grammar as the core for this in-depth cognitive linguistic investigation, namely, construction grammar, word grammar and metonymic grammar. Cognitive grammar has a comprehensive meaning construction that will serve as a backdrop for much of the consequent discussion in this book. This chapter includes a preliminary discussion of figurative use of language, which will be integrated into the cognitive grammar as a unified framework of meaning construction within medical promotional discourses. Chapter 3 talks about the research method, data collection. Within the context of empirical and usage-based accounts, the reliance on cognitive grammar involves the use of introspection and argumentation based on a series of analyses of naturally occurring data. Chapters 4, 5 and 6 deal with "Metonymic PoV in Promotional Discourses of Anti-Cancer Medicines", "Force Dynamics in Promotional Discourses of Online Treatments" and "Grounding Grammar in Promotional Discourses of Medical Treatment Appliances" respectively, concerning word construction at three different linguistic levels. Chapter 7 summarizes the main cross-cultural findings of the present study and proposes a new orientation for future research in cognitive linguistics, social linguistics and cross-cultural communication studies. In addition, this chapter also presents a more exhaustive account of linguistic discussion on cognitive grammar which operates at various levels of meaning description identified in commercial medical discourses. Furthermore, the book explores the cross-cultural differences related to the combination of cognitive operations and discourse analysis in the creation of given meaning effects.

1.7　Summary

This book is a supplement to the author's previous work *A Cross-cultural Study of Commercial Media Discourses: From the Perspective of Cognitive Semantics*. This volume further shows how usage-based, data-driven and classic bottom-up approaches should be integrated with one another, and how the combination of them allows the analyst to address the cross-cultural linguistic differences which might frame different kinds of cognition. The contributions of this book highlight challenges related to both discoursal research methods as well as applied linguistic studies for cognitive linguistic analyses and generation. Because both types of approaches have their strengths and weaknesses, their combinations have been used and will continue to be used for both linguistic and natural language process (NLP) purposes in medical communication fields. In addition, the findings of this book can provide cross-cultural and empirical evidences for professional communication and AI language training within the commercial fields—at least in relevant areas, as well as for future empirical validation in applied linguistics and cognitive sciences. Thus, the author conducts a usage-based cognitive grammar approach to commercial discourses in a specific professional field to provide evidences to people in professions in the selection and determination of the nature and organization of linguistic systems in communication.

Chapter 2

Cognitive Linguistics and Cognitive Grammar

With the development of psychology and cognitive science in recent years, linguistic researchers are showing growing interest in the relationship between language and human minds, promoting the rise of cognitive linguistics and making it a popular and fruitful research area. As a research approach, cognitive linguistics provides theories and methods that can be applied in various fields of linguistic study and it can also be combined with other disciplines to explore the cognitive mechanism and cognitive foundation of human minds underlying the language use. Based on the previous studies, the book analyses the medical promotional discourses (about medicine, online medical treatment and medical appliances) from the perspective of cognitive grammar, specifically, on PoV, force dynamics and grounding, to provoke the cognitive models, meaning constructions and grammar rules and their linguistic representations and disciplines.

2.1   Development of Cognitive Linguistics

In the past decades, substantial progress has been made in understanding the neurobiology of perception, appraisal, attention, memory, and cognition from a linguistic perspective. Among them, cognitive linguistics is a kind of language research method and paradigm which is different from traditional grammar, structure, and generative grammar in philosophical basis, language view and research methods. Most traditionally, Lakoff and Johnson (1999) put forward the Embodied Philosophy and clarify its position of the philosophical foundation of cognitive linguistics, echoing the concept of "experientialism"

(Lakoff & Johnson 1980) and summarizing three principles of the Embodied Philosophy as the embodied mind, the cognitive unconsciousness, and metaphorical thought (Wang 2002, 2006), which upholds the importance of human mind and bodily experience in communication. In other words, during communication, communicators produce meanings and understand others based on their thoughts and experiences. As Croft and Cruse (2004) see it, the major hypotheses and theories of the cognitive approach to language in the 1980s represent a response to the pioneering approaches to syntax and semantics, namely, the generative grammar. Based on experientialism, cognitive linguistics holds that language is the product of the interaction between the internal factors of human beings and the external factors of the object world. Cognitive linguistics emphasizes the role of human experience and cognitive ability (rather than absolute objective reality) in language use and understanding, holding that there is no so-called meaning independent of human cognition, nor objective truth independent of human cognition (Goldberg 2009). Language is not a closed and self-sufficient system, but an open and dependent one. It is the result of a combination of objective reality, social culture, physiological basis, cognitive ability and other factors (Zhao 2002).

Generally, cognitive linguistics holds that language not only reflects the cognitive process and results of the real world, but also is a tool for people to know about the world. Among them, Schumann (1994) holds that the brain is the seat of cognition, that cognitive processes are neural processes, and that, in the brain, affect and cognition are distinguishable but inseparable. The idea that concepts are embodied by our motor and sensory systems is popular in current theorizing about cognition. Embodied cognition accounts come in different versions and are often contrasted with a purely symbolic view of cognition (Chatterjee 2010). According to the cognitive view of experiential realism in cognitive linguistics, the cognitive subject (a person) always chooses a certain position when he/she understands the object (objective thing), that is, perspective. The choice of perspective is the embodiment of subjectivity, which directly affects the subject's understanding of things. Cognitive linguists believe that we conceptualize the world through the use of conceptual devices like metaphor, metonymy, and image schema, which are motivated by our human embodiment, reflected in cognitive structures. In other words, cognitive mechanisms are motivated by human embodiment (Lakoff & Johnson 1980). As Brisard (2002) suggests, cognitive linguistics holds that people's perspective of observing things is closely related to language expressions: (1) the choice of perspective has an important impact on semantic structure; (2) language expression has different structures due to different perspective choices. People generally have regular location systems, which are part of their encyclopaedia knowledge system. For unconventional perspectives, they need to refer to different horizontal/vertical systems and take different perspectives. Their brains' abilities to transform have important impacts on semantic structure while they communicate with others. No matter what their actual perspectives are, the speakers can understand them from different perspectives, so as to express the same situation appropriately (Zhao 2002). For instance, the reporting verb is a typical example to illustrate the above mentioned theory: the discourse writer can use reporting verbs to quote others' opinions, and he/she unconsciously adds his/her cognition and attitude to these verbs and, thus, the verbs carry emotions that will influence readers, especially those who possess different viewpoints against the writers (i.e. Chinese readers and American authors who have an adversarial attitude towards China). However, many scholars analyse cognitive frames to illustrate the features of human beings' cognition construction. Fillmore (1985: 223) introduces the concept of "frame", defining it as "a specific unified framework" of knowledge or coherent schematizations of experience. A frame provides necessary background concepts for understanding the meaning of any concepts. For instance, a "dining frame" is involved while understanding the meaning of "eat", a concept that indicates the relationship between eater and food, together with relevant tools and environmental settings. All of the above components form the "dining frame" and comprehension of any concept therein requires the participation of at least part of other concepts. Frame semantics, therefore, upholds that in one's mind, understanding of the entire frame is the prerequisite for comprehending any concept therein (Li 2008).

In addition, scholars also explore the different cognition mechanisms at discourse level. Discourses or texts, in this sense, serve as the carrier of human minds. The encoding and decoding mechanisms in the discourses require the employment of various cognitive mechanisms like reasoning, inferring, and conceptualizing. Understanding the meaning of the discourse involves both decoding of the surface and literal meaning of the words, and it also involves the identification of the "embodied mind" beneath the discourse.

Cognitive research tools such as construction grammar and metaphor have been widely applied in analysing various linguistic phenomena involved in cognition. Dancygier and Sanders (2010) attempt to understand more clearly the applicability of cognitive frameworks used so far by analysing the textual choices and genre differences to shed light on the relationship between form and meaning from the perspective of cognitive linguistics. From their study, it can be found that some discourses, like poetic discourses, are shaped to some extent by metaphor, but other meaning-construction mechanisms, such as grammatical structures and semantic frameworks, are equally important.

In terms of textual studies of linguistics, text coherence is the core of relevant research. The mechanisms of text coherence include explicit coherence and implicit coherence. Coherence, as van Dijk (1977) argues, is a semantic feature of texts which depends on the relationship between the interpretation of each single sentence and other sentences. The explicit mechanism of coherence lies in the information structure and cohesive devices of a text, while the implicit mechanism rests with the relationship between language and psychology, culture and social cognition. Holtgraves and Yoshihisa (2007) allege that many processes are essential to social cognition like attribution, perception, and stereotypes, involving language in some manner.

One of the difficulties in textual studies is to understand the complex relationship between context and text (W. Z. Lu & Y. Lu 2006). In order to demystify the complexity, it is necessary to interpret how the textual representation relates to the deeper conceptual representation, that is to describe the link of discourse structure and the psychological activities involved in information processing. Li (2013) delves into textual coherence with reference to the concept of cognitive frame by comparatively exploring Chinese and American texts. He proposes that discourse interpreters should construct their own thoughts based on the concepts activated by words, phrases, clauses and paragraphs in the text within the micro, meso and macro cognitive framework.

2.2 Semantic Studies of Cognitive Linguistics

As Langacker (1987a) professes, "What distinguishes cognitive semantics from other research branches of semantics is that cognitive semantics claims that meaning is a cognitive phenomenon, which needs to be understood and analysed from the perspective of cognition" (Yang 2020: 16). Lakoff and Johnson (1999) believe that cognitive semantics studies the reasoning of human beings, and it is the description of conceptual structure which is the product of a cognitive process. They insist that there is no semantics independent of cognition, and no objective truth independent of human cognition. Talmy (2000:4) proposes that "cognitive semantic research studies conceptual content and its organization in language, the nature of conceptual content, and language organization in general". In this way, cognitive semantics puts the meaning of language at the center of its studies. The dialectical relations between human mind, language and embodied experience play important roles in the studies on cognitive linguistics. From a cognitive perspective, linguists focus on the relations among language, cognitive model, knowledge structure, even the relationship with nervous system and mentality. In order to elucidate these relations, semantic studies are placed in a pivotal position in cognitive studies (Wang 2002), and it remains its great popularity and influence in the field of linguistics study.

Cognitive semantics concerns categorization, conceptualization and so on. For instance, concerning conceptualization, Fillmore (1982, 1985) connects linguistic semantics to the encyclopaedic knowledge that one holds, while Lakoff (1987) highlights an "idealized cognitive model (ICM)" to illustrate the relationship between a semantic domain and some external background experiences. In this field, Talmy (2000) analyses the relationship between conceptualization and meaning itself to observe how the semantics structure is affected by conceptualization, and introduces schematic category, force dynamics and perspective point, and so on. Such a focus attends semantic domain, ranging from spatial relations (e.g. Kreitzer 2009) to human emotions (e.g. Jing-Schmidt 2007). As for categorization, starting from levels of categorization developed by Lakoff (1987), Croft and Cruse (2004) study the functions of conceptual categories, followed by Aski (2001) on phonological split, by Schubert (2014) on conversational strategies, by Gogichev (2016) on idiom semantics, and by Stibel (2006) on vitality from a cross-disciplinary study of categorization. These studies achieve huge development in cognitive linguistics.

Within more specific contexts, Zeng (2008) identifies six basic features of cognitive semantics. The first feature is that meaning is equal to conceptualization in cognitive model. Language meaning is the mapping of linguistic expressions to cognitive or psychological entities. Evans and Green (2006) reckon that the meanings expressed by language units are just subsets of concepts. Since semantic structure is conceptual, and semantic understanding is a process of conceptualization, so meaning decoding is a process of cognition construction which may be involved in cognitive concepts, such as conceptual blending. The second feature is that the main basis of meaning is perception. Cognitive structure in our brains is directly or indirectly related to the perceptual mechanism of our body, which means the meaning base of language is at least partly rooted in human perception. The third feature is that semantic components are based on spatial or topological objects. Gärdenfors (1995) points out that the conceptual schemes, which are to represent meanings, are not symbol systems with syntactic structures, but are based on geometric or spatial configuration. The fourth feature is that the main attribution of cognitive model is image schema, and its transformation mechanism is metaphor and metonymy. The fifth feature is that semantics is the basis of and partly determines syntax. Cognitive semantics holds that semantics, as the main component of language, appears in the form of perceptual representation and has existed long before the complete evolution of language, which is very different from generative linguistics that syntax is autonomous and can operate independently of semantics and semantics is a secondary additional feature of language. The last feature is that concepts have a prototype effect. Wu and Chen (2004) suggest that conceptual category is the most basic factor of human cognition, because semantic categories are the reflection of the external world.

2.3   Cognitive Studies of Media Discourses

Discourse analysis has developed into an interdisciplinary field since 1960s. Media discourse is one of the imperative media through which people use to get information from the society and the world, serving as the source of human knowledge, attitudes and ideologies (van Dijk 1998). Generally, the language used in media articles needs to be concise, impartial and objective. However, in real-life media, news discourses confront social, institutional and individual factors that could make the objectivity of journalists trying to pursue, for instance, self-cognition, institutional stance, individual attitude, and even political trends. Being a practical genre of discourses, news discourse has attracted great attention and discussion from scholars who have devoted various definitions to news discourses. van Dijk (1998) defines news discourse from the perspective of social context, illustrating news discourse as the main source of human knowledge, attitudes and ideologies. Sharing the similar concept, Fowler (1991) describes news discourse as a social practice and product that discourse reporters have produced based on the news topics they have chosen to reflect their newsworthiness criteria.

Among sociolinguistics studies, cognitive sociolinguistics appears as an emerging field in media studies, casting light on the application of cognitive sociolinguistics analysis in societies. Proposed and explicated by Kristiansen and Dirven (2008), cognitive sociolinguistics comes into being with a hope of furnishing a cognitive explanatory framework for those linguistic utterances under social backgrounds, whose ultimate goal is actually to set up a mental model for the interrelation between society, individuals and institutions. Yet, this burgeoning inter-discipline, which researches on the social implication of cognitive linguistics, still has a long way to go before being widely acknowledged by academia, so is the analytical method of cognitive sociolinguistics.

Generally, cognitive linguistics in media discourse aims to reveal how the cognitive process of journalists influences news productions and projects news interpretations. Such an approach is concerned with how people construct language and meanings by choosing different semantic and linguistic devices. CL offers a paradigm towards the interpretation of epistemology and ideology embedded behind semantic preference in news discourse, which includes theories like CBT (Cognitive Blending Theory), metaphor theory, frame semantics and metonymy as well, stressing the sociological and psychological aspects. For quite a long period of time, metaphor and CBT have been the two main theories that attract the most research interests. van Dijk (1985, 1988, 1998, 2006) introduces linguistics research and cognitive analysis into media discourse. He puts forward three levels of ideology and discourse: social analysis, cognitive analysis and discourse analysis. He argues that discourse analysis is linguistic analysis based on the social context, and proposes that discourse analysis is in fact ideological or epistemological analysis (van Dijk, 2008). He suggests a model that differentiates "we" and others, such as "the journalists" and "the readers". Such a model exerts influence on how people behave, including speaking and writing. The overall stance and base are in line with van Dijk's findings and contribution in this area.

Cognitive-oriented discourse analysis has been emerging as cross-disciplinary with other methodologies and serves as complementary in media discourse studies. For instance, socio-cognitive approach proposed by van Dijk (2008) and cognitive-oriented critical discourse analysis. Yang (2020) presents a cross-cultural cognitive study of commercial discourses, showing the possibility of the fusion between cognitive linguistics and CDA. Moreover, critical metonymy analysis has been receiving amounting attention (H. Zhang & T. W. Zhang 2012). The above studies do shed light on the efficient comprehension of news discourses for discourse consumers or newsreaders but few of them dig into the closer relationship between overt language and covert cognition, especially in the contexts of different cultures (Yang 2020). Yang (2020) explores the complex yet thought-provoking correlation between overt language and covert cognition by focusing on contrastive analyses of metaphors, image schemas and stance markers in commercial media discourses by analysing their linguistic applications, lexical devices and personal experience, along with their embodied mechanism. She argues that the combination of cognitive studies and media discourse analysis offers comprehensive and rewarding insights into the cross-cultural research of both cognitive actions and linguistic behaviour reflected in news reports and highlights the correlation between the use of wording and cognitive construction in discourses, which broadens the scope of discourse analysis, cognitive linguistics, applied linguistics and sociolinguistics. Her findings unveil the vitality of empirical semantic study and thus enrich the diversity of cognitive linguistic studies of media discourses.

2.4　Studies of Cognitive Grammar

Cognitive Grammar holds psychological realities in high regard in linguistic description (e.g. Langacker 2004). Traditional approaches to grammar have paid more attention to language forms, structures and the description or interpretation of the internal relationship at different levels, such as the phoneme, morpheme, syntax. However, the approaches to grammar based on cognition lay full emphasis on the functions of cognitive subjects, the cognitive methods and conceptual systems. Cognitive approaches to grammar focus directly upon the linguistics system. Although Taylor (1995) puts forward that the study of cognitive semantics is within the framework of "cognitive grammar", Geeraerts (2005) and Talmy's (1988) claim on cognitive grammar is more broadly compatible with Langacker's approach (1987a, 1991) which focuses on meanings of language. For instance, within cognitive grammar, spatial thinking and language influences how people think, memorize and reason about spatial relations and directions. In the last decade, substantial progress has been made in understanding the neurobiology of perception, appraisal, attention, and memory. For instance, at lexical level, Abutalebi and Clahsen (2015) hold that cognition might reasonably be conceived as consisting of the perception of lexical stimuli, the emotional appraisal of the stimuli, attention to the stimuli, representation of the stimuli in memory, and the subsequent use of that information in behaviour. The brain stem, and limbic and front-limbic areas, which comprise the stimulus appraisal system, emotionally modulate cognition, therefore, in the brain, emotion and cognition are distinguishable but inseparable. Therefore, from a neural perspective, affections are integral parts of cognition.

At semantic level, Langacker (1987a: 189) claims that "basic grammatical categories such as noun, verb, adjective, and adverb are semantically definable". He believes that any language expression will activate several cognitive domains, called the complex matrix. CG defines the typical members through the prominent domain. He defines a noun as a thing or an entity, which is profiled in a domain. A verb is a process profiled in a temporal domain and others like prepositions, adjectives, and adverbs are profiled in a temporal domain. The difference between a process and a temporal relation is the different ways of mental scanning. The former is sequential scanning through which we observe each stage of an evolving scenario one by one. The entire conceptualization is dynamic, and its content is always changing. The latter is summary scanning, through which we observe all aspects of a scene cumulatively, gradually building an increasingly complex concept.

It is argued that meaning is determined by the way we construe and the content that the expression represents by using semantic features or semantic primitives when describing the meaning of words. In other words, the producing or understanding of an expression involves the speech itself together with the certain manner the event described. Construal is defined as the inherent capability to conceptualize and represent a given scenario through alternate methods (Croft & Cruse 2004). The interpretation of an expression can vary based on the observer's viewpoint. This concept encompasses five dimensions: specificity, background, perspective, scope, and prominence. In terms of depicting our perceptions of the environment, language production offers us multiple options. For instance, the degree of granularity with which we describe an object (specificity) and the element of a composition we select to emphasize (focus) are decisions within our control.

One of the construal systems at lexical level is force dynamics, which is responsible for conceptualization. Object's movement or change in their being or motion leads Talmy (1988) to develop force dynamics theory which involves two entities, the agonist, and the antagonist. Typically, the agonist associates a force keeping it in place or a force tending it towards motion while the antagonist exerts a force contrary to that associated with the agonist. He argues that deontic modals are metaphorically a kind of force. Further, based on force dynamics theory and metaphor theory, Sweetser (1990) compares the deontic and epistemic modality with forces and claims that the absence or presence of a physical barrier (e.g. "can" and "may") or compelling force (e.g. "must") in the socio-physical world is mapped onto the absence or presence of reasoning or compelling forces in reasoning. Langacker (2008) considers English modal verbs which lack tense and person markers as grounding elements, who reveals that "modal verbs as grounding elements import the notion of potency directed toward an event's occurrence" (p. 304). Root modals relate to notions like obligation, permission, intention and ability and their modal force is manifested in the realm of social interaction. The locus and result of the potency are internal to the conceptualizer's knowledge. Comparatively speaking, Langacker's (2008) notion of grounding element adds contextual elements, producing a more explanatory model for native speakers' perception, experience and representation of things and speech events.

At textual level, the approach of cognitive grammar (CG) to discourse analysis primarily emphasizes the mental mechanisms involved in the formation and understanding of discourse, which investigates the manner in which linguistic expressions represent specific interpretations of discourses and, conversely, examines the interpretations' impacts on the reader's pre-existing knowledge and capacity to decode the physical, social, and linguistic elements of the presented expressions (Langacker 2008). Put differently, CG seeks to understand the processes through which texts are constructed, comprehended, and assessed.

Initial explorations in discourse studies utilizing CG framework have predominantly investigated its role in shaping construal within literary discourses, as evidenced by research conducted by Harrison et al. (2014), Stockwell (2009), and Yan (2021), among others, including Hart (2014) and Zhang & Luo (2017). Similar to how lexical elements convey meaning, the interpretation of a statement is determined by both its conceptual content and the specific manner in which the content is construed. For instance, Stockwell (2009) identified construal as a crucial linguistic mechanism for generating meanings within literary texts. Yan (2021) delved into the grammatical features of the novel "The Handmaid's Tale," highlighting how cognitive construal approaches, such as scanning and specificity, elucidate diverse readings of the fiction's themes from psychological and ideological standpoints. By examining media discourses, Hart (2014) also emphasized the significance of functional grammar, multimodal grammar, and CG in uncovering the ideological dimensions of discourses within socio-political frameworks, arguing that cognitive processes integral to language comprehension are inherently linked to visual perception. Moreover, Harrison et al. (2014) broadened the application of CG in discourse analysis through the incorporation of concepts like the action chain, reference point model, profiling, and compositional path in the study of contemporary fiction. From a critical perspective, Zhang and Luo (2017) pursued a critical cognitive examination of strategic intelligence discourse through a CG lens, further elucidating CG's applicability in the analysis of intelligence discourse.

2.5   Word Grammar

Word Grammar (hereafter abbreviated as WG) is a theory created and formalized by Richard Hudson in the 1980s as a branch of cognitive grammar studies, which is one of the most important components of cognitive linguistic studies, and a very hot topic of applied linguistic studies as well. It is a theory of language structure and receives its name for its rejection of phrase structure, and it centres on the linguistic fields from syntax to semantics, morphology, sociolinguistics, historical linguistics, cognitive linguistics, language learning and language processing (Hudson 1984). That is, unlike other constructional theories, WG eschews phrases. Traditional grammar takes "phrase" as the basic unit in syntactic analysis to reflect meanings, while WG uses "word" as the only unit to establish semantic networks based on dependent relations. As Hudson (2010) put it, WG is also based on the assumption that language, and indeed the whole of knowledge, is a network, and that virtually all of knowledge is learned. It combines the psychological insights of cognitive linguistics with the rigour of more formal theories. Besides, WG is part of the very old linguistic tradition of dependency grammar. Within this framework, syntactic structure is based, not on the part-whole relationships of phrase structure, but on the dependencies between pairs of words. Basically, the principles of WG rest on cognitive science, shedding more light on the process of humans' cognition in language. Furthermore, WG provides a new method and tool for exploring the nature of language and its way of syntactic analysis can be applied in grammar studies and teaching practice.

Regardless of the "practical difficulty", there are still theories that corroborate the collaboration of CL and semantics and lexical typology, e.g. WG. WG is such a combinative and coherent theory that integrates a wide range of theories with cognition into one, with an initial attempt to build a generative version of Systemic Grammar, sharing properties both from Systemic Functional Grammar and cognitive science (Hudson 2010). WG is a theory which has received its name for its rejection of phrase structure (Hudson 1984), but its focus on language has broadened from syntax to semantics, morphology, sociolinguistics, historical linguistics, language learning and language processing since then. In an overview of WG by Droste and Joseph (1991), the most obviously non-standard feature of WG is that it deals with the whole of syntax without referring to anything but words—the notion "phrase", "clause" and even "sentence" play no part in a WG grammar. According to WG, dependency relations between words are basic and constituents grouped around words are derivative, whereas phrase structure grammar assumes that the relation between constituent structure and dependency is the other way around.

Another noteworthy characteristic of WG syntactic structure is that grammatical relations are also taken as basic, rather than as derivative. Moreover, grammatical relations are viewed as organized hierarchically. So in this way, WG integrates two well-established grammatical ideas, namely dependency and grammatical relations. Features are in fact used in WG syntax, but only in the narrowly restricted domain of morpho-syntactic features. WG is a model of syntactic analysis based on the following assumptions.

1) Except in coordinate structures, the largest syntactic unit is the word.

2) There is no formal distinction between statements in the grammar about individual words and statements about classes of words.

3) A grammar is a set of propositions defining relationships among entities, the most important of these relationships being those of INSTANTIATION, COMPANIONSHIP and COMPOSITION.

In brief, WG rejects the traditional and persisting distinction between grammar and lexicon. WG postulates that Language is a conceptual network (Hudson 1984) in which each network element—whether a word or a word property—possesses connections of various sorts, both semantic and syntactic, to one or more other elements. Hudson (2007) proposes the "new" WG, which differs from his two previous expositions (Hudson 1984) first and foremost in its expanding embrace of everything experimental psychology has determined about linguistic and other cognitive processing, especially in its incorporation of the processes of "spreading activation" and "default inheritance" as the prime sources of dynamism and efficiency in language networks. Regarding language as part of human knowledge, Hudson (2010) sees the importance of laying a cognitive foundation for WG, and introduces WG from three aspects: its theoretical bases on cognitive science, its major arguments in linguistics, and its up-to-date explanations for various linguistic phenomena related to English. He, therefore, explains a number of commonly accepted ideas and facts in related disciplines, such as activation, attention, chunking, default inheritance logic, episodes, frequency effect, long-term memory and working memory, network, parallel distribution processing, priming, prototypes, schema, scripts, selective memory etc. When presenting these ideas, Hudson (2010) adds his own perspective to them. He argues that: (1) Relations are concepts, and can be classified into open-ended taxonomies through "a" hierarchy just the same way as entity concepts can; (2) Default inheritance (DI) should be monotonic and apply to exemplars only; (3) Landmarks (Langacker 1987b) must combine "prominence" and "nearness" to be suitable. Hudson holds that the best landmark is the one that keeps the best balance between prominence and nearness; (4) Mental activity goes beyond activation; (5) Binding is the third basic activity type in our cognitive network, besides activation and node-building. Holding his ground firmly, Hudson applies the above ideas to explaining linguistic phenomena, particularly those related to English, so as to achieve a merge of the general insights of cognitive science into how our minds work with the enormous amounts of detail that linguists analyse (Yue & Liu 2011).

2.5.1　PoV grammar in cognitive linguistics

Many cognitive linguists believe that language is embodied in bodily experience (Croft & Cruse 2004; Lakoff & Johnson 1980, 1999). One crucial experience for human is the spatial relation around us. Since childhood, we have experienced something close to or far away from us, and we have distinguished left and right, up and down. All these spatial relations give us a sense of direction and distance, providing us with perceptions of the world. Language is deeply influenced by spatial relations and we hold the ability to construct and represent things from a specific viewpoint or perspective, which is embodied in our language system. As Langacker (2008: 75) suggests, many grammatical constructions invite the conceptualizer to construct the scene from a particular point of view. He proposes that one component of the viewing arrangement is a presupposed vantage point. In the default arrangement, the vantage point is the actual location of the speaker and hearer. The same objective situation can be observed and described from any number of different vantage points, resulting in different construals which may have overt consequences. Many expressions undeniably invoke a vantage point as part of their meaning (arguably, all expressions do).

Inspired by Lim's (2004) visual-grammatical model and many cognitive discoursal theories that focus on spatial relations in discourse like the Discourse Space Theory (DST) and Proximization Theory (Chilton 2004; Cap 2006; Yang 2023), Hart (2014, 2015) advocates the application of PoV grammar in linguistic discourse, which delves into the spatial relation, especially the point of view in the linguistic discourse and its application. Before identifying PoV in linguistic discourse, Hart (2015: 247) clarifies two concepts in PoV grammar. For one, event space (ES) refers to "a mental space set up for the currently described event in the unfolding discourse"; it is a place where the conceptualization takes place. For the other, basic space (BS) is a grounding space in which the conceptualizer's point of view is determined (Radden & Dirven 2007; Dancygier & Sweetser 2012; Hart 2015). According to Hart (2014, 2015), three fundamental variables exist in PoV grammar, namely anchor, angle and distance. Every variable is endowed with four values: X_1 to X_4 for anchor, Y_1 to Y_4 for angle, Z_1 to Z_4 for distance.

2.5.1.1 Anchor

Anchor relates to the horizontal viewpoint from which one perceives the scene. Cognitively, anchor decides which side the conceptualizer chooses to stand behind and shares the same perspective with. Grammatically, the change of anchor takes place in asymmetrical and reciprocal transactive clauses as well as distinct voices and information structures (Hart 2015). The variable of anchor in PoV grammar is represented in Figure 2-1.

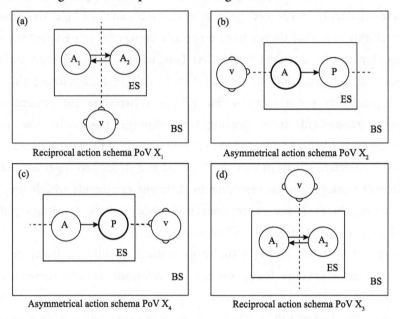

Figure 2-1　Anchor in PoV Grammar (Hart 2015: 248)

Note: A stands for agent, P for patient and V for viewer. Throughout this book, ES means event space, and BS means basic space.

In Figure 2-1, PoV X_2 takes the perspective of agent whilst PoV X_4 takes the perspective of patient. We tend to construct the asymmetrical actions, i.e. unidirectional action from the two perspectives, since one entity will exert effects on another when one conducts an asymmetrical action. For one thing, by using active or passive tenses, linguistic expressions allow the agent or the patient to be the subject of the sentence, and decide which participant shows up and is represented in the viewer's mind first so as to put the specific participant in a rather prominent and close position to the viewer. This participant will then share the same perspective with the viewer or reader. For another thing, in PoV X_1 and X_3, the viewer adopts a rather fair anchor point as a bystander; yet disparities still exist for the fact that people have the habit of viewing things from left to right at a horizontal level, which results in the difference between anchor point X_1 and X_3 in terms of the participants' sequential order of entering the viewer's eyes. Grammatical constructions like reciprocal transactive clauses are generally endowed with such anchor points.

2.5.1.2   Angle

In contrast to the anchor, an angle relates to the vertical spatial relation concerning perceiving a scene, which can be closely related to nominalization and certain types of metonymies like WHOLE FOR PART and COLLECTION FOR SINGLE ENTITY since these linguistic representations use generalized terms to form the intended meaning. Two of the four angle points are portrayed by Hart (2015), which are shown in Figure 2-2.

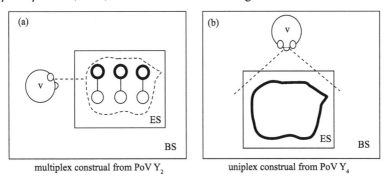

Figure 2-2   Angle in PoV Grammar (Hart 2015: 253)

We can imagine that when we perceive a scene from the bird's eye, i.e. PoV Y_4, many details will be omitted because we are directly above the scene in which we may only be able to observe its surface or outline, leaving many other details unobservable. In contrast to Y_4, Y_2 provides a relatively equal position to observe the scene where details are presented clearer. Generally speaking, angle results in the alternation in plexity and number (Hart 2015). The former concept refers to whether the perceived scene is conceived as a complex comprising a number of individual elements or as a simple whole. The latter concept, on the other hand, refers to the singularity and plurality of the involving nouns in the linguistic representation (Talmy 2000; Hart 2014, 2015).

2.5.1.3 Distance

Distance is the third variable in PoV grammar which decides how much the portion of a scene can be seen by the viewer, or which portion is placed in the viewing frame of the scene. According to Hart (2015: 253), a viewing frame contains the conceptual content that is currently the subject of the viewer's attention in the proceeding discourse. Figure 2-3 presents models for four values of distance.

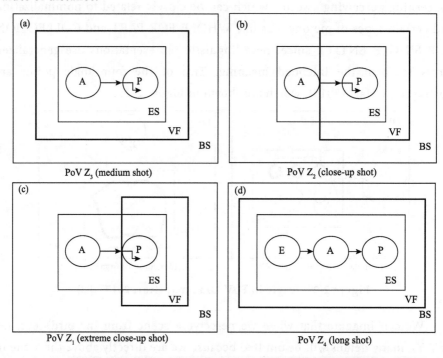

Figure 2-3 Distance in PoV Grammar (Hart 2015: 254)

Note: In the figures throughout this book, VF means viewing frame.

From value Z_1 to Z_4, the distance between the viewer and the scene becomes larger as a larger portion of the scene is entering the VF. That is, Z_4 represents the largest distance. The E circle in (d) of Figure 2-3 refers to the preceding events of the action; the distance is so far that the preceding event can also be observed while viewing the current scene. In (a)-(c) of Figure 2-3, the arrow's extension into the patient suggests that the action has changed the state of the patient, which can only be observed at a relatively close distance. Hart (2015) argues that linguistic phenomena that limit the range of VF include the agentless passive voice, the absence of causation circumstantial clause and certain nominalization.

Based on the above analysis of the three variables in PoV grammar, Hart (2015) puts the three variables within one model to represent the whole PoV system. See Figure 2-4.

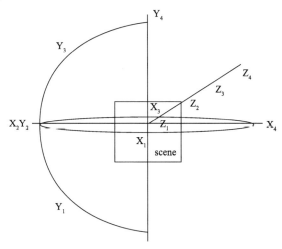

Figure 2-4 PoV Grammar (Hart 2015: 244)

As can be seen, the scene is measured by three variables which allow the viewer to choose any point to perceive the scene. In reality, countless points in every axis provide limitless points of view, but only some of them (X_1-X_4, Y_1-Y_4, Z_1-Z_4) are picked up and represent different viewpoints. The selected points of view then lead the readers to build up construction from a specific perspective; different points of view generally produce different interpretations in the same sentence.

For the purpose of comprehending the Anti-Cancer medicine promotional discourse comprehensively, it would be of great significance to observe the point of view from which the sentence is constructed. Based on the above analysis, point of view is endowed in the grammatical construction of linguistic representation, and it influences how the meaning is expressed. Considering that most people are unfamiliar with medical discourse or business discourse, a different point of view may form a completely different understanding and cognition toward the discourse itself or even related phenomena.

2.5.2 Force dynamics in word grammar

Word grammar is proposed by Ruiz de Mendoza and his collaborators (e.g. Ruiz de Mendoza & Baicchi 2007; Ruiz de Mendoza & Mairal 2008; Ruiz de Mendoza & Galera 2014), aiming at systematically explaining the intrinsic relationship between construction and human cognitive models, and reveal how different kinds of conceptual pattern interact to yield complex meaning representations, such as force dynamics. Force dynamics represents a semantic field that encapsulates the interactions between entities and forces. This semantic field infiltrates various layers of language, proving its relevance not only in describing physical actions like leaning or dragging but also in articulating psychological impulses such as desires or compulsion. Besides, the framework of force dynamics extends into the realm of discourse analysis, exemplified by scenarios where Speaker A concedes to Speaker B, illustrating a dynamic interplay of forces. Originally conceptualized as an evolution of traditional causality notions, it segments causality into finer elements, incorporating actions of permitting, obstructing, and assisting. The pivotal figure in this domain, Talmy (1985, 1988, 2000), methodically explored how force dynamics inform the creation of meaning within language. His research demonstrates the linkage between cognitive and sensory experiences with the tangible world, alongside the interplay between our physical bodies, sensory perception, and external physical entities engaged in forceful interactions, including the application, opposition, impediment, and resolution of forces. He believes that force is part of our conceptual structure. Force is ubiquitous and can be expressed through grammar and lexicon in language structure. The force-dynamics system encodes the "naive physics" of our conceptual system (our intuitive rather than scientific understanding of force dynamics), and has implications not only for the expression of relationships between physical entities, but also for abstract concepts such as permission and obligation. Force-dynamics system well elaborates on the relationship among the concepts like exerting force, resisting to force, overcoming resistance, performing physical actions that exist in the force-dynamics formula. The main idea of force-dynamics system lies in that there are two force-exerting entities and they act mutually (interaction) and exist in language expressions.

Talmy (2000) classifies force contained in language expressions (mainly single sentences) into three categories: physical force, psychological force and social force. Physical force is the most basic type of human body experience, while psychological force and social force are metaphorical extensions based on physical force. Talmy's (1988, 2000) force-dynamic theory includes some fixed elements and three main patterns. A basic force-dynamic schema includes four factors, as seen in Figure 2-5. In the study of force dynamics, the primary entity under consideration is termed the Agonist, while its opposing entity is known as the Antagonist (Ant, symbolized by a concave figure). Ago has its own force tendency which can either be shown or be overcome by an opposing force, usually referred to as Antagonist (Ant), which is able to exert forces that are contrary to the forces of Ago. The description of Ant depends on the effect of its force exerted on Ago. "b" refers to the intrinsic force tendency of force entities. Arrowhead means the tendency is toward action, while big point means the tendency is toward rest. "c" refers to the balance of strengths of two force entities, "+" means stronger entity, "−" means weaker entity. "d" refers to the resultant of force interaction, arrowhead means a tendency of action after the interaction, while big point means it is a rest tendency.

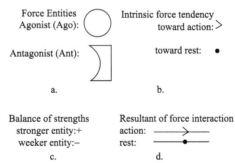

Figure 2-5　Force-dynamic system elements (Talmy 2000: 414)

As Yang et al. (2016) put it, the outcome of the force-dynamic scenario depends on both the intrinsic tendency and the balance between the forces. For instance, "The door cannot open" can be force-dynamically represented in Figure 2-6 (see pattern d in Talmy 1988: 55).

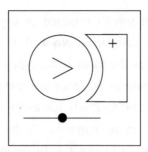

Figure 2-6 Force-dynamic schema of "The door cannot open"

Utilizing these basic components of force dynamics theory, complex force-dynamic patterns can be examined to achieve rewarding results. Talmy (2000) puts force dynamics in a broader cognitive and semantic context. In his view, the basic idea of this subject is that there is a fundamental difference between the closed type (grammar) and the opened type (lexical) language. The motivation for this distinction is that language uses certain categories of concepts to construct and organize meaning, while other categories are excluded from this function. For example, he comments that many languages label the number of nouns systematically, but the colour of nouns is different. Force dynamics is considered to be one of the closed concept categories, along with generally recognized categories such as quantity, aspect, emotion, and evidence. Aspects of force dynamics have been incorporated into the theoretical frameworks by researchers, such as Johnson (1987) and Jackendoff (1990). Force dynamics plays an important role in several recent accounts of modal verbs in various languages (Boye 2001). Other applications of force dynamics include use in discourse analysis (Talmy 1988, 2000) and morphosyntactical analysis (cf. Langacker 1999). Over a few decades, force dynamics theory has been employed in psychological area, teaching area and forensic linguistics. However, up to now, there is little discussion on the change of perception of hearer from the perspective of force dynamics and psychology knowledge. Hence the change of perception of hearer which is based on force dynamics theory can be a direction of further research.

2.5.3　Grounding grammar

Grounding theory is first proposed by Langacker (1991) in his work

Foundations of Cognitive Grammar and further develops into nominal and finite clause grounding by Langacker (2008) who emphasizes that the use of grounding elements contributes to the connection between the object (entity) or event (process) and the cognitive scene in the mental space of speech event participants. In other words, the speaker relates an entity or process to the current speech event in such a way that the hearer gains cognitive access to or mental contact with the entity or process. The essence of this theory is how the relationship between the entity or process and the speech event affects the form and meaning of an expression.

Grounding theory reflects the conceptualizing relationship between the conceptualizer and the conceptualized, shown in Figure 2-7. Langacker (2008) regards the speaker and the hearer as S (subject of conception), and the profiled content as O (object of conception). In the full scope of awareness where everything falls in the visual field, those elements that are not salient or at the margins of awareness in the discourse will be present offstage. Then S is subjectively construed. For example, the word "tomorrow" only evokes the time reference but does not emphasize it explicitly. The focus of attention is unconsciously directed to the intended object at the onstage region with maximal objectivity. Then O is objectively construed.

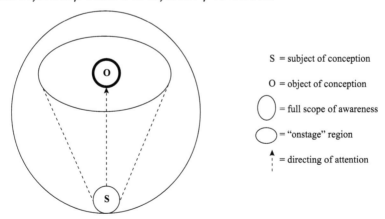

S = subject of conception

O = object of conception

◯ = full scope of awareness

◯ = "onstage" region

▲ = directing of attention

Figure 2-7 Subjective and objective construal (Langacker 2008: 260)

A nominal or a finite clause profiles a grounded instance of an object/a thing, or process type. It is crucial to distinguish type and instance of that type in order to understand grounding. Broadly speaking, a nominal is like a noun

profiles an object/a thing; a clause that includes a verb profiles a process (Langacker 2008). A noun designates a type of object/thing, and a verb a type of process. Without grounding, a noun or a verb merely refers to a type of object/thing, or process. Considering the expression "girls like boys", "girls" or "boys" refer to a type of object with indefinitely many instances but fail to be figured out as any particular instances. The lexical verb "like" specifies a "process type" in which there are countless situations as there are different boys and girls. A specific process type can be defined when its participants are elaborated as individuals. By contrast, through grounding, the expression "the girl likes the boy" refers to a particular instance of this type. By grounding "girl" and "boy" with the definite article, the speaker directs hearers' attention to a specified context. Through clausal grounding, the instance is situated at present, not in the past or the future.

2.5.3.1 Grounding predication

In Cognitive Grammar, the term ground refers to the discourse context in which language is used. Specifically, a ground consists of a speech event, the participants in the speech event and the immediate circumstances (place and time of speaking). As Langacker (2008) claims, grounding is the process whereby grounding predications (also including grounding elements like determiners) function to link a profiled thing or process to the ground.

According to Langacker (2002), there are three characteristics of grounding predications. First, grounding predications are a set of highly grammaticalized elements. For example, articles and tenses are highly grammaticalized and lose their independent functions. They are chosen as the final step in forming a full nominal or finite clause. In other words, grounding elements help to designate an instance of a type, forming a nominal or finite clause. Second, grounding predications are epistemic in nature. Their specification of the relationship between the ground and the designated thing or process specifies some very basic notions which are "epistemic" in nature, such as time, reality, immediacy, and identification. Third, grounding predications put the grounded entity onstage instead of the grounding relationship and the ground. For example, the demonstrative "this", does not profile the relationship of identification and of proximity to the speaker, but profiles the object/thing related to the ground, which is its conceptual referent, that is, "the object/the thing" or "the process".

2.5.3.2 Grounding classification

Based on the literature on grounding studies, the present research classifies grounding into clausal, tense and modal grounding.

1. Clausal grounding

The essence of a finite clause is how the relationship between the designated entity and the ground or situation of speech, affects the clause's form and semantic meaning. Grounding predicates need to turn verbs into finite clauses. A simple verb can merely specify a process type, while only a finite clause can designate a grounded instance of that type.

The clausal grounding elements are tenses (v, v+"-ed", v+"-s/es", etc.) and modals (e.g. may, can, will, shall, must, might, could, should, would), which specify a particular instance. That is, the grounding predicates serve the function of locating the speech event before, during and after the time of speaking, or indicating a potential situation. According to Langacker (2008), only tenses and modals have epistemic values, which can realize the grounding functions, while perfective, progressive and passive aspects only highlight a certain aspect of the grounded event process, namely completed, in progressive, or passive aspects. Grammatically, both the tense and modality are obligatory in a finite clause, while the perfective, progressive, and passive aspects are optional.

2. Tense grounding

Tenses as grounding predications include the present and past tenses (future tense being marked by modals). The opposition between the present and past tenses is best analysed in terms of whether a process is immediate to the ground or distant in either time or reality. The degree of our epistemic certainty of the event is positively correlated with the position of the time of the event relative to the time of speaking. That is, the closer the occurrence time is to the speaking time, the greater the cognitive certainty of it. Specifically, Langacker (1987b) characterizes that PRES (present) indicates the occurrence of a full instantiation of the profiled process that precisely coincides with the time of speaking; PAST indicates the occurrence of a full instantiation of the profiled process prior to the time of speaking.

3. Modal grounding

The absence and presence of a modal in a clause indicates whether the process belongs to reality (where the ground is located), or is out of the reality, or is the potential of the reality. Main modals include "may, can, will, shall, must, might, could, would, should". The modals "might, could, would, should" indicate the non-immediacy of the epistemic judgment itself. For example, by using "might" rather than "may", the speaker indicates that the judgement implied from "may" is not sanctioned by his own immediate circumstances. According to Langacker (2008), modals unleash a kind of force to impose the trajector tending towards an action, and since the modals are grounding predications, they are offstage and subjectively construed, as shown in Figure 2-8. Only the target of the force or the grounded process or entity is left onstage.

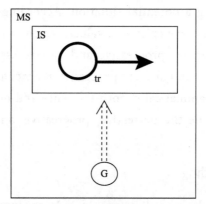

Figure 2-8   Grammaticalized modals (Langacker 2008: 304)

Note: In the tables and figures throughout this book, MS means maximal scope, IS means immediate scope, Tr means trajector, and G means ground.

2.6   Summary

The literature on cognitive grammar (CG) has been briefed above. CG is a newly-developed linguistic area that still needs constant supplements and refinement. At present, cognitive linguistic scholars have carried out relevant research into the analysis of CG from different perspectives. The research into this area combined with other fields, such as syntax, morphology, cognitive linguistics, and grammaticality in cognitive grammar construction, has yielded many achievements. Some scholars even manage to apply this theory to language teaching and language acquisition. Obviously, more about CG needs to be further developed. CG may have a facilitative role to play in language studies. Additionally, there are few analyses of CG from the perspective of sociolinguistics and empirical research. This book can be considered as a systematic study on cognitive grammar for future research orientations. It is believed that with constant research, the exploitation of CG will be invariably updated.

Chapter 3

Contrastive Discourse Research and Design

Contrastive discourse analyses are very fruitful in communication studies, which investigate discourses within different cultures in order to smooth intercultural communication in which both discourse writers and readers combine their knowledge, experience and cultural heritages to construct their cognition and understanding of the world. In doing so, both writers and readers make crucial links between their cognition construction on the one hand and the discourse that frames that cognition on the other hand. As Lü (1982) puts it, only by making contrast could we see the commonalities and particularities of various linguistic manifestations. Therefore, the so-called theory of linguistics is actually a contrast between languages, which is the scientific conclusion drawn from a contrastive analysis of various languages in the world.

3.1   Contrastive Discourse Studies

The rise of contrastive discourse studies has benefitted from the development of two disciplines, that is, contrastive linguistics and discourse analysis. The cross-cultural analysis of discourse construction patterns started in the mid-1960s, with a paper by Kaplan (1966) as the landmark, *Cultural Thought Patterns in Inter-Cultural Education*, which mainly focused on English as a Second Language (ESL) students with various cultural backgrounds from different nationalities. With five different paragraph expansion types, the study shows that Anglo-European texts go with linear development. By contrast, textual paragraph development in Semitic is based on a series of parallel coordinating clauses; emphasis of prose in Eastern languages is often placed at the end; prose, in Romance and Russian, allows for a certain degree of digression. With the related research results on the rise, his views have created a new field of contrastive discourse, which does not fail to fascinate other scholars.

From the 1970s to the 1980s, researchers around the world conduct studies on contrastive discourse analysis mainly from the following two aspects: i) discussion and examination of the feasibility of Kaplan's (1966) hypothesis; ii) possibility and necessity of expanding the scope of comparative discourse analysis. At this stage, scholars have studied the issues in multiple languages. Hartmann (1980) compares discourse construction patterns in Japanese and Western languages; Eggington (1987) examines the contrast between English and Korean; Connor (1987) contrasts discourse in English, Finnish and German texts; Singh and Kachroo (1987) discuss differences in discourse cohesion between Hindi and English. The above-mentioned contrastive discourse studies shed light on language cohesion and discourse construction. In addition, Hartmann (1980) and Krzeszowski (1989) emphasize the importance of parallel texts when discussing methods for contrastive discourse analysis.

After the 1990s, as a large proportion of influential results have been published one after another, the way of contrastive discourse research gradually broadened. Based on the textual linguistics theory of Beaugrande and Dressler (1981), Martin (1992) proposes a macro-discourse description framework in an attempt to deal with contrastive rhetoric research in practical discourse. Furthermore, with contrastive discourse analysis, rather than limiting it to the comparative study of the structure of discourse, he argues that other factors should be taken into account in the production of discourses. Swales (1990) provides an interesting model for defining discourse types and discourse communities in contrastive discourse study, arguing that it compares discourses written for similar purposes in similar contexts. Pankow (1992) reckons that, by comparing television news in Germany, Russia and America, we can see that people's thinking patterns affect their interpretations of language use and the layout of the texts in different cultural environments and contexts.

For the time being, the language barrier lies more in the application of language than in the language itself. R. Scollon and S. Scollon (1995, 2000) put forward the concept of discourse systems. They assume that cultural differences should not be analysed in terms of language systems but discourse systems as the basic unit and more consideration should be given to the discourse system of each region, country and nation.

The contrastive discourse analysis began in the early 1980s, with Qian's (1983) article "A Comparison of Some Cohesive Devices in English and Chinese" published in *Foreign Languages*. With the advancement of comparative linguistics and discourse analysis in China in the 1990s, the study of comparative discourse has made gratifying progress. For instance, Wang and Li (1993) investigate the way Chinese students were thinking in their English writing and compare it with native English speakers, and Li (1998) reflects on the phenomenon of Kaplan's (1966) use of biased language in contrastive discourse rhetoric from a critical perspective, and puts forward the possibility of avoiding this situation in *The Value Orientation of Contrastive Discourses in English and Chinese Discourse Studies*. In the meantime, the emergence of a large number of related books also reflects the rapid development of comparative discourse research in China. For example, in *Contrastive Linguistics*, Xu (1992) discusses the research methods of contrastive linguistics, and makes a specific comparison of the cohesion and coherence of discourse, which plays an important role in promoting the development of contrastive research; Xiong (1999) conducts the research from the perspective of cognitive grammar, and compares English and Chinese anaphoric phenomena from the perspective of cross-cultural communication in his work; "A Contrastive Analysis of Semantic Structures in English and Chinese" (Lu 1999) takes semantic theory as the framework with self-built corpus. The paper deals with the similarities and differences in the semantic structure of the two languages, providing a juicy corpus resource for scholars of contrastive discourse research.

In the 21st century, the contrastive study has taken a new step, and the subject has turned to develop in the direction of specific and same writing-style discourse comparison. For example, Xu (2004) conducts a comparative discourse analysis on the similarities and differences between

English and Chinese texts, offering a discoursal perspective for the cross-cultural communication study. Ma (2002) reviews the general situation of contrastive text research by Chinese writers in the past 20 years since the 1980s, which has important reference significance for future studies. Xu (2004) emphasizes the importance of social and cultural contexts in the analysis of contrastive texts in his article called "On Cross-Cultural Contrastive Discourse Analysis". From the perspective of translation, Xu (2005) provides rich examples by comparing the Chinese and English texts and analysing the different ways of realizing interpersonal meaning in the two texts of *The Scholar* (《儒林外史》)and its translation. It further explores the deep cultural connotation as well as the value orientation of writers and translators. Yang (2009) makes a thorough inquiry into the thematic structure and pragmatic phenomenon in communication, enriching the cross-cultural discourse analysis. On the basis of move structure and social cognitive research framework, Cheng and Yang (2017) believe that the similarities and differences in values affect the journalists' cognition of a specific event in a certain context to some extent through a comparative analysis of the smog-related news.

　　Contrastive discourse studies around the world as well as profiling a number of researchers that represent each geographical area and cultural tradition, and researchers study cross/inter-cultural discourses from multiple linguistic perspectives, at different levels and even from cross-disciplines. Although compared with foreign countries, Chinese scholars are late starters in contrastive discourse analysis, they have gained excellent achievements after the 1990s. Since the 21st century, the research has turned to a more in-depth and specific field. Generally, the disciplinary boundaries and questions of identity have been common concerns for researchers involved in the field of business communication in particular, the field in which some researchers who are interested in business discourse are active. As Hatim (2001) puts it, doing discourse analysis without a contrastive base is as incomplete as contrastive analysis without a discourse analysis base, and discourse analysis going hand in hand with contrastive analysis will result in a better understanding. The contrastive research between languages and linguistic phenomena, is usually termed as contrastive linguistic analysis, or contrastive linguistics.

　　The profound connotation of contrastive analysis has attracted so much attention from both Chinese and foreign linguists that they attach quite an importance to contrastive studies of languages. Their works are often endowed with high academic and practical values by exploring their own languages on the basis of other languages or through the contrastive analysis of different languages so as to reveal the similarities and differences between language applications, such as grammar and word patterns, in projected cultures. The method of contrastive analysis has been employed in far-flung fields within linguistics, ranging from translation, language teaching, especially second language acquisition, to cross-cultural research. For instance, at the discourse level, Wallmach and Kruger (1999), based on the examination of problem-solving strategies adopted by student translators, argue that the differences of languages and cultures push to broaden the concept of translation to a much more practical and functional level where translation adaption and reformulation are given much consideration, enlightening on the translation advancement based on the contrastive analysis. With regard to contrastive linguistic analysis in second language acquisition, Lardiere (2009) touches upon the selection and assembly of certain features in second language acquisition by comparing the assembling and expressing ways of features in plural-making in English, Korean, and Chinese. She claims that processing certain lexical items of a second language demands that the language learner reproduce the features into the second language in the way in which they are composed in the first language, and draws a conclusion with some general thoughts on the role of Universal Grammar in a second language acquisition.

It is not hard to spot from previous studies that contrastive discourse analyses are often applied in cross-cultural research, drawing inspiring conclusions about different cultures for participants to better communicate in multi-cultural settings. That is, the contrastive discourse studies devoted by former scholars fall within the scope of comparing cultural differences or answering the question of "what is different", while as for questions like "what leads to cultural differences" and "how those differences are formed", few studies have yet been conducted. Therefore, it is of great necessity for this book to touch upon the complicated cognitive and mental issues in driving such cross-cultural variations based on contrastive discourse analysis.

Nevertheless, current contrastive discourse analyses from cognitive perspectives do shed light on the efficient comprehension of news discourse for discourse consumers, or news readers, such as Yang's (2020, 2023) researches. However, these studies are mainly restrained in the categories of lexicology, semantics, pragmatics, and common linguistics, paying less attention to the syntactic or grammar levels and thus failing to dig into the close relationship between overt language and covert cognition, especially under different cultural contexts. Considering this, the author of this book aims to make a contrastive study of Chinese and American medical discourses from cognitive grammar theories, hopefully revealing the different thinking patterns intertwined with cognitive and cultural factors between Chinese and Americans and helping the smooth promotion of medical products.

3.2   Contrastive Linguistic Studies on Media Discourses

The profound connotation of contrastive linguistic analysis has attracted much attention from both Chinese and foreign linguists, whose analyses are often endowed with high academic and practical values by exploring their own languages and another language through contrastive linguistic analyses and cultural studies. For instance, a contrastive analysis of media discourse in English and Chinese newspaper is launched by R. Scollon and S. Scollon (2000) who observe and conduct research on different ways of employing quotations, which embarks on the development of cross-cultural contrastive media discourse analysis. Grounding on the news data sourced from *The Washington Post* and *The Daily Times* of Nigeria, Chaudhary (2001) investigates the significance of cultural variability in selecting international news, who examines the possibility of whether news focuses on reports about individuals or groups, and whether such emphasis being equipped with positive or negative tones in the U.S. and Nigeria. By contrasting the news reports from the U.S. and Nigeria, Chaudhary (2001) proposes a preliminary assertion that collective needs, values, and goals foreshadow the individual needs, values, and goals, which provides a brand new perspective into contrastive analysis on cross-culture studies.

In two decades, plentiful contrastive studies on metaphors in media discourses have been carried out. Linguists (e.g. Charteris-Black & Ennis 2001; Charteris-Black & Musolff 2003; Yang 2020) are interested in analysing linguistic metaphors and conceptual metaphors in financial reports in newspapers by comparing English and other European languages. They find that many similarities exist in conceptual metaphors while subtle differences do appear in terms of linguistic expressions. For instance, Spanish news reports prefer to take metaphors of psychological mood and personality as their base, while the English counterparts go for nautical metaphors (Charteris-Black & Ennis 2001). From a pragmatic approach, Charteris-Black and Musolff (2003) prove that metaphors have impacts on opinions because they emphasize the ornamental function of metaphors. Semino (2002) also conducts a contrastive analysis of metaphorical patterns used in texts to describe "the euro" in Britain and Italian newspapers. Apart from identifying similar source domains of metaphors such as JOURNEYS, CONTAINERS, and BIRTH shared by English and Italian, Semino (2002) suggests that to back up different opinions of monetary union, novel metaphors are used as rhetorical devices in both languages. In another comparative study of metaphors in English and Russian, Wang et al. (2013) are interested in conceptual metaphors and metaphor frequency analysis from the perspective of pragmatics. Their results reveal many cognitive similarities in conceptualizing economic crisis since the English and Russian share basic metaphorical structures. While in terms of the frequency of metaphors and the linguistic expressions of corresponding metaphors, certain differences do emerge that more metaphorical expressions are used in English texts. In addition, this research also interprets crisis metaphors from universal and cultural-specific perspectives. The finding points out that metaphors in Russian articles demonstrate more diversities and pragmatic forces than those in English articles. In the cross-linguistic comparisons of the MARKET metaphors, Chung (2008) lays out both "MARKET" metaphors and collocates of "MARKET" (in reference to grammatical roles) used by people of the three different languages at a grammatical level. By discussing the similarities and differences, Chung (2008) reveals that varied source domains indicate diverse grammatical roles for "MARKET", who also suggests that in terms of "MARKET" the perspectives of people speaking the same language can be inferred by making metaphor semantic meaning analysis and their relationship with grammar.

To associate with feelings and psychology, researchers target the metaphorical expressions in the area of emotion—anger in news reports. By means of comparing English and Chinese emotional expressions of anger, anger expressions in Chinese appear to be more related to "HOT GAS" metaphor, and the cause of heat, namely fire, being closely linked to internal organs, while the English notion of anger is usually expressed as "HEAT" and "HOT FLUID" (Dirven et al. 2012). The existence of various culture-specific realizations of conceptual metaphor in cognitive linguistics has embarked on the metaphorical cognitive contrastive linguistics. *A Contrastive Study on Basic Emotion Conceptual Metaphors in English and Persian Literary Texts* written by Mashak et al. (2012) attempts to explore the universal and unique metaphorical conceptualization pattern in English and Persian, mainly around feelings like happiness, anger, sadness, fear and love. Through categorizing and comparing hundreds of emotive metaphorical expressions, they highly support the concept of universality in the conceptualization of the two cultures, though some cultural differences are acknowledged.

At semantic level, Fukuda (2009) examines the function of metaphors in creating technical terms for different phases of a business cycle in Japanese and English. He reckons that metaphors change together with the phrase of a business cycle facing each economy, what's more, the verbal, adjective and adverbial terms only exist in U.S. mechanical metaphor and that the number of metaphorically used adjectives and adverbs in English is larger than those in Japanese. Yang (2020: 88), by comparing Chinese and English metaphors in business (High Speed Railway, HSR) news discourses, argues that metaphorical representations in news reports are characterized by both cognitive universality and cultural relativity. The motivation behind similar metaphorical expressions in English and Chinese news discourses can be attributed to universal cognition patterns. Given that bodily experiences cannot be singled out from the particular cultural surroundings they take place, it is anticipated that there should be differences among the conceptual metaphorical systems in varied cultures.

Overall, there are various contrastive analytical methods applied to news discourse through a literature review which does shed light on the efficient comprehension of news discourse for discourse consumers, or news readers. However, those contrastive studies are mainly restrained in the categories of semantics, pragmatics, and general linguistics, paying less attention to the cognitive level and thus failing to dig into the close relationship between overt language and covert cognition, especially under different cultural contexts. Considering this, the author of this book aims at making a contrastive linguistic study of Chinese and English media discourses themed on medical products based on cognitive grammar theories, namely, metonymy, lexical grammar and WG.

3.3   Contrastive Studies on Cognition Construction

Namely, decoding discourse is equivalent to the process of constructing cognition, or called cognitive processing. With regard to the construction of cognition in discourses, cognitive linguists frequently use the concept of "cognitive frame" to analyse the cognition construction contained in discourses. The main source of human cognition of things is people's experience and perception of objective things (Holmes & Stubbe 2003). Theoretically, contrastive analysis regarding language structure does not study the relationship of language in the real world, but the relationship inside the different units of language. However, cognitive linguistics holds that language not only reflects the cognitive processes and results of the real world, but also is a tool for people to know about the world. The contrastive linguistics, as a way for people to know about the world, needs cognitive linguistics to identify the similarities and differences in cognitive mechanisms between countries and in their language systems; meanwhile, its research goal of peeking into the cognitive mechanisms behind language through studying of linguistic phenomena can be truly realized. Thus, cognition-based contrastive studies between English and Chinese have been flourishing in recent years, touching upon a range of fields. Searching the Internet, the author finds that contrastive cognitive linguistics can be extended to foreign language teaching, teaching Chinese as a foreign language, language acquisition, translation, dictionary compilation, literature research, natural language processing and other fields. Wen (2002) also puts forward several research methods in contrastive cognitive linguistics, which are synchronic and diachronic, micro and macro, static and dynamic, qualitative and quantitative, inductive and deductive. As a result, comprehending how people organize their knowledge and reproduce it in mind has been a long-term interest of cognitive linguists.

Many scholars do not solely conduct contrastive research on cognition, but also through analyses of language phenomena explore the cognition mechanisms behind them. The current contrastive research directions on the cognitive and psychological mechanisms of two languages are dialyzed. For instance, Zhang (2006) conducts a contrastive cognitive study on English and Chinese double-object sentences at syntactical level, showing that the construction and its verbs are involved in different ways of interaction, while at lexical level, Peng and Bai (2007) find that conceptual metaphor and conceptual metonymy serve as an effective cognitive tool to understand human emotion through the cognitive research on Chinese and English newly-coined affective word "angry". Through the contrastive study of new words, Peng and Bai (2007) find that the new words are not only conducive to testing the previous cognitive mode, but also to embodying the growth of cognitive mode. More comprehensively, Yang (2020: 149) proposes that the cognitive process in different linguistic cultures is to some extent a mental mechanism whose purpose is to derive a semantic representation from a linguistic expression. Different discourses and semantic patterns in fact emerge out of cognitive activities. As for linguistic applications, Abutalebi and Clahsen (2015) examine the role of bilingualism in cognitive development and aging, analysing whether bilingualism provides any "specific" benefits to general cognitive abilities that are covered under the label of "executive function", i.e. processes that manage and control other cognitive activities, such as attention, visual perception, and switching between languages.

Accordingly, both cognitive linguistic studies and cross-cultural studies place language or discourse in a central position, delving into its relationship with underlying values and ideologies for cognitive construction. For one, linguistics studies necessitate cross-cultural comparisons in order to connect linguistic phenomena to cultural issues and enhance the practical significance.

For another, the insufficient analysis of language use is, to some extent, a major deficiency of cross-cultural studies considering that language is an indispensable part of culture.

3.4 Contrastive Discourse Research Design

The author applies a critical approach to the present study by combining discourse study, sociolinguistics study, cognitive study, pragmatics study and grammar study of a specific professional communication context, in which critical thinking concerns the disciplined process of conceptualizing, analysing, interpreting, synthesizing and evaluating the linguistic elements related to cognitive grammar in medical promotion texts as the dominant discourses in Chinese and English.

The texts analysed are mostly retrieved from the official websites of authentic and top Chinese and American medical companies, such as pharmaceutical factories, medical devices production and treatment organizations. In this book, the author chooses promotional discourses of Anti-Cancer medicines, online medical treatment and coronary stent for the present analyses on cognitive grammar. The Chinese data consists of 30 texts in three different medical fields respectively issued by Chinese and American medical companies from the year 2012 to 2022.

The author adopts both quantitative and qualitative analysis on the textual data collected by the aforementioned procedure, utilizing the webpage-crawling tool and corpus tool to collect the data for a contrastive analysis. By virtue of the webpage-crawling tool (Octopus) and corpus tool (AntConc), the data gathered for the present analysis involves more than 120,000 words in the corpus. First, the research classifies the lexical devices and categorizes them for qualitative study by decomposing certain verbs and nouns lexically, semantically and syntactically. The words are identified by the corpus tool, not taking into consideration the frequencies but identifying and annotating both the word itself and its collocations in the sentence. Statistics of different groups of data are used to reveal the linguistic preferences and thinking patterns. Then, the meanings and interpretations in the discourses are decoded afterward applying qualitative analysis. Being combined with the interpretations, the cognitive construction, processing and perception behind the numerical preferences and thinking patterns thus are unfolded in each language system. In addition, a comparative study is utilized in dealing with cross-cultural cognitive differences and similarities to complete the expected analytical procedure on cognitive grammar studies. The research procedure follows a consistent pattern.

Firstly, the author has closely examined the 30 texts respectively in three different analytical fields and manually identified the lexical devices, such as verbs, modals, and metonymies, presented in the data according to the linguistic categories in both Chinese and English analysed in Chapters 4, 5, and 6. The distribution and frequency of each category are identified and calculated respectively. Then the author examines the construal process by taking a closer look at the locus of the potency, the target the potency directed, and the agent carrying out the potential acts. A contrastive summary of the results derived by quantitative and qualitative methods can generate valuable cognitive patterns in two languages and provide cross-cultural insights for communication studies and marketization studies.

Secondly, the cognitive grammar related to lexical devices, such as the model of "modals + V", will be identified and analysed in discourses based on cognitive grammar, unveiling the mental representation of how lexical devices function to influence the cognitive construction and discourse comprehension. For example, as for modal verbs and their cognitive analyses, the profiled verbs will be first classified in view of Langacker's (1987b) distinction of perfective and imperfective processes designated by verb applications. Then cognitive models employed in English and Chinese discourses are sketched to reveal what kinds of potential acts discourse producers intend to project and how discourse writers employ modals to make their statements more acceptable so as to construct the public cognition.

Thirdly, a discussion will follow the contrastive analysis to justify the cognitive differences revealed by the comparison of the cognitive mechanism reflected from the overt language use in English and Chinese promotional discourses, in the hope of obtaining cognitive and cross-cultural implications therein.

3.5 Summary

Researchers who study discourse ask many different kinds of questions, and they need many different theoretical and methodological tools to answer them. What the author uses and describes in this book is a methodological tool that is useful, or is potentially useful, in the disciplinary and interdisciplinary inquiry of cognitive linguistic studies. Cognitive grammar used for the present discourse study, as the author has described in this section, is rigorous to the extent that is grounded in the closest possible attention to linguistic, contextual and contrastive details, i.e. the author conducts a contrastive analysis of cognitive representation in medical communication field, which will be certainly associated with customer's merchandising behaviour and company's marketing strategies. Such an interdisciplinary study is systematic to the extent of cognitive grammar and it encourages the author and other researchers to develop multiple explanations before they argue for one. Thus, interdisciplinarity of this present study is thus not just an attractive feature of discourse analysis but a central fact about cognitive science, because discourse analysts, including the author herself, have often drawn on multiple disciplines besides linguistics for possible ways of explaining things, and the world as well.

Chapter 4

Metonymic PoV in Promotional Discourses
of Anti-Cancer Medicines

In recent years, China and America have witnessed great improvements in the field of cancer medicine and treatment, with pharmaceutical companies emerging and developing rapidly. However, they might not share the same perceptions and cognition with regard to illness, medicine, treatment and other medical issues, creating noteworthy cognitive and cultural differences. Hinged on the theories introduced in Chapter II on PoV grammar, the present study analyses the metonymic expressions and their grammatical PoV constructions in the Anti-Cancer medicine promotional discourses.

4.1　Introduction

Based on Radden and Kövecses' (1999) and Croft and Cruse's (2004) definitions of metonymy, the author examines the sixty pieces of discourses in both the Chinese and English corpus, identifying all the linguistic items which employ one concept to replace another within the same domain/domain matrix or ICM for the sake of providing mental access to a relatively inaccessible concept. The qualified item will then be marked as metonymy and sorted according to the metonymy type. In addition, both the source and the target of each metonymy will also be identified so as to prepare for classification and further analysis.

4.2 Data for Metonymic PoV Studies

4.2.1 Data

The data analysed in the chapter is retrieved from news published on official websites of world famous pharmaceutical companies where reliable information about Anti-Cancer medicines can be found. The first step of data collection is to select those companies that produce or sell the Anti-Cancer medicines. To begin with, the author uses the search engine Google and Baidu and search the key words of "American pharmaceutical/medical company", "Chinese pharmaceutical/medical company", etc. Most of the selected companies generally have broad service coverage and large business scale, enjoying good reputation and positive influence. Based on the above criteria, the author finally selects fourteen pharmaceutical companies.

The second step is to collect the discourse. While browsing the official websites of these companies, the author notices that all of these websites are set with "media" or "news" buttons ("媒体动态" or "新闻中心" in Chinese) on the main page. The corresponding pages provide information about industrial highlights or product development of the company. Reports about the introduction of their Anti-Cancer drugs and the development or promotion of new drugs are exactly the kind of discourse that this chapter probes into. Therefore, the author screens the report on the "media" and "news" pages of each chosen company, randomly selecting 60 texts related to Anti-Cancer drugs, including 30 pieces in Chinese and 30 pieces in English, to form a Chinese and English corpus for this study. Each of the above-mentioned texts is numbered; Chinese texts are numbered from CT1 to CT30 while English texts from ET1 to ET30. Table 4-1 shows relevant data.

The data presented in Table 4-1 dates from Jan. 2016 to Aug. 2019. All the six companies from which the English data is retrieved are American companies. During data selection, the author excludes several influential pharmaceutical companies like Swiss companies Novartis, Roche and German company Bayer. Guided by the research aim of studying Anti-Cancer medicine promotion in China and the U.S., the author is forced to leave these companies out for the reason that they are not Anti-Cancer professional manufacturers despite their great industrial influence.

Table 4-1   Chinese texts and English texts

Types	Company Name (Abbr.)	Amount of Texts	Text Numbers	Types	Company Name (Abbr.)	Amount of Texts	Text Numbers
CTs	复星医药 Fosun Pharma	7	CT1-CT7	ETs	Pfizer	9	ET1- ET9
	恒瑞医药 Hengrui Pharma	5	CT8-CT12		Sandoz	1	ET10
	绿叶制药 Lvye	4	CT13-CT16		Bristol-Myers Squibb	6	ET11-ET16
	誉衡药业 Yuheng	4	CT17-CT20				
	药明生物 Yaoming	3	CT21-CT23		Merck	5	ET17-ET21
	正大天晴 Zhengda tianqing	3	CT24-CT26		Abbvie	4	ET22-ET25
	和记黄埔 Heji huangpu	3	CT27-CT29		Amgen	3	ET26-ET28
	丽珠医药 Lizhu	1	CT30		Lilly	2	ET29-ET30

Note: In the tables and figures throughout the book, CT means Chinese text, ET means English text, and Abbr. means Abbreviation.

4.2.2 Research method

By studying metonymy in the Anti-Cancer medicine promotional discourse and delving into the similarity and disparity of metonymic expressions in both Chinese and English corpora and their corresponding implications, the author adopts both qualitative and quantitative research, supplemented by the descriptive and comparative analyses.

According to Given (2008), quantitative research in social sciences adopts statistical, mathematical, or computational techniques to study observable phenomena. He suggests that quantitative data is any data that is in numerical form such as statistics, percentages, etc. In this study, the quantitative approach is embodied in the author's measuring the frequencies and percentages of different metonymies that appeared in the corpora. As mentioned earlier, metonymy displays human beings' metonymic thinking, demonstrating people's cognition and values. It would be evident that the more frequently a metonymic type appears, the more important the underlying value is. Meanwhile, after analysing all the points of view adopted to construct the metonymy by the discourse producer, the author calculates the frequencies of different points of view in both Chinese and English discourses to figure out different preferences therein.

Qualitative research, combined with descriptive research, is used to answer research questions 1 and 2, which probe into metonymy types, the manner of its embodiment and the points of view that discourse producers employ to construct the metonymy. On the one hand, descriptive research, which addresses the "what" question, i.e. describes characteristics of a group of people or a situation being studied (Shields & Rangarajan 2013), is utilized to identify and classify the metonymy in the linguistic data. On the other hand, qualitative research is a scientific method of observation to gather non-numerical data, answering "how" and "when" a phenomenon occurs (Babbie 2014; Berg & Lune 2016). Therefore, instead of focusing on the question of "how much", it probes into the implications and characteristics of the research objectives by analysing specific examples of the metonymy in the two corpora. The analytical tools of PoV grammar will facilitate the analysis on metonymy at syntactic level and semantic level.

4.2.3 Analytical procedure

In this chapter, comparative research, together with both quantitative and qualitative analyses, is adopted to dig into the cultural differences between China and the U.S. and the corresponding implications concerning metonymies and PoV. In light of Peirsman and Geeraerts' (2006) classifications of metonymy, the next step is to classify metonymic representations into different categories in reference to the source and target of the metonymy. According to their classifying method, each of the categories is named by the format of "source & target" which is borrowed as the category name of the metonymy analysed in this chapter. After sorting the metonymy in the data, the author calculates the frequency and percentage of each category so as to range them numerously and analyse them respectively.

Then, the author analyses the metonymy at a sentence level from the perspective of PoV grammar, a theory put forward by Hart (2015). He employs a three-dimension model which contains three parameters, namely anchor, angle and distance, to analyse the point of view of the grammatical construction of metonymy. The metonymic representation identified in the first step will then be examined grammatically, which delves into the point of view the discourse producer adopts to construct the metonymy, indicating different representation manners to satisfy the objective in mind. Then, to semantically decode the cognitive process of understanding those metonymic categories, metonymies are analysed by virtue of the PoV. The author employs this model to explain how the angle provides mental assessment to the target, building up the cognitive connection between the metonymies and their grammatical uses. By virtue of the above analysis, the author draws a conclusion about the cognition behind the metonymic representation appearing in the Anti-Cancer medicine promotional discourse, which, the author argues, closely relates to the values and ideologies about medicine promotions.

After the analyses of metonymy grammatically and semantically, the author compares the frequencies of the adopted point of view and metonymy of each type, figuring out the preferences of metonymy used in both Chinese and English texts for interpreting the promotion patterns and values embodied in Sino-American Anti-Cancer medicine promotional discourses. Finally, after the cognitive analysis and cross-cultural comparison of the point of view adopted to construct metonymy and the cognitive process of decoding different metonymy types, the author attempts to summarize the cultural differences between China and the U.S., yielding implications concerning the promotion of Anti-Cancer medicines.

4.3   Metonymy as a Lexical Unit in Cognitive Grammar

In other words, people's bodily experiences offer part of the fundamental basis for language and thought. Metonymy is regarded as a figure of speech, but now it is one of the basic ways of thinking for people to understand the nature as they think and talk about daily events metonymically (Gibbs 1999). It is considered as a physiologically oriented type of embodiment (Maalej & Yu 2011; Zhang et. al. 2015). Though metonymies play an important role in people's daily communication, they have been eclipsed by substantial discussions on the role of metaphors (Handl & Schmid 2011). Metonymy application is a key issue for cognitive grammar study with its focus on a specific type of lexical unit. Many scholars have devoted themselves to the study of metonymy for decades, putting forward influential approaches to explaining this linguistic phenomenon. As Lakoff and Johnson (1980) put it in their work, metonymic concepts structure our language by the way of constructing our thinking modes and behaving patterns. Metonymies are grounded in our experience and the grounding of metonymic concepts is more obvious than other figurative concepts, encompassing physical and causal associations.

Traditionally, metonymy is viewed as a figurative tool used to realize the rhetorical function of text, which is analysed in the category of figure of speech, just like metaphor which is also first defined as a kind of figurative expression (Lakoff & Johnson 1980). Ancient philosopher Aristotle identifies four types of metaphor, yet three of which are later viewed as metonymy by modern linguists, namely Genus for Species, Species for Genus and Species for Species (Mahon 1999). The commonality of the traditional view of metonymy lies in the appreciation of its rhetorical function with three similarities: (i) metonymy is a figure of speech; (ii) metonymy involves the word substitution; (iii) metonymy takes root in proximity and closeness.

The figurative view of metonymy dominated the philosophical and linguistic study of metonymy for years. Many researchers focus on the aesthetic and figurative functions of metonymy, defining it as "an ornament" or "a figure" to substitute one word with another (Givón 1978; Preminger & Brogan 1993), who point out a common feature while using metonymy. As the replacement or change of word(s) describing an entity or event, metonymy is mainly studied at lexical and rhetorical levels. Al-Sharafi (2004) supports this argument by claiming that the figurative function of metonymy is based on the proximal relation between related words, suggesting that it is the proximal relation that causes the alternation of words. The major problem with a traditional view to the metonymy is that it fails to explain the cognitive process in decoding metonymy or metonymic expressions. The traditional view has not considered or explained how metonymies are embodied in discourse cognitively, or how metonymic expressions are represented in human mind. To answer the above questions, linguists gradually turn to a cognitive view of metonymy. Metonymy, nevertheless, is an intriguing topic in cognitive linguistics and metonymic concepts are one of the most basic characteristics of cognition. Like metaphor, metonymy is grounded in human life and our everyday experience but in a less rhetorical way. It's extremely common for people to take one easy-to-perceive aspect of something and use it to stand either for the thing as a whole or for some other part of it. A straightforward definition of metonymy is that metonymy is a cognitive process whereby we use one entity, process, or event to stand for another related entity, process or event, which means it has primarily a referential function. But, meanwhile, it is not a mere referential device. Metonymy also serves as providing understanding. The specific part we pick out determines the aspect of the whole we are to focus on (Lakoff & Johnson 1980).

4.3.1   Definitions on metonymy

With the development and popularization of cognitive science, especially cognitive linguistics, more efforts of studying conceptual metonymy have been made, yielding abundant outcomes in this field. Cognitive linguists argue that metonymy functions as more than a rhetorical or an aesthetic device. Metonymy is also closely related to human cognition and represents certain kinds of conceptual patterns. The exploration of the relationship between metonymy and human mind/conception forms the main body of the cognitive view of metonymy (e.g. Croft 1998; Lakoff & Johnson 1980; Panther & Thornburg 1998, 1999, 2007; Radden & Kövecses 1999; Talmy 2000).

Initially, Lakoff and Johnson (1980: 36) specifically devote their efforts to the portrayal of metonymy, who define that metonymy "has primarily a referential function, which allows us to use one entity to stand for another". This definition makes an evolutionary progress in the metonymy study. In this definition, they first associate the concept of "cognitive domain" with metonymy, stressing the important role human cognition plays in using metonymy. To illustrate the cognitive basis of metonymy, Lakoff and Johnson address this issue by using the term "contiguity" which, in a way, agrees with the idea of proximity and closeness suggested by the traditional view of metonymy, but entails new content in their interpretation. They believe that the basis of conceptual metonymy is physical or causal relations (Lakoff & Johnson 1980), which views the proximity of the words and their meanings solely as the basis of metonymy. Another two important components of metonymy identified by them are the vehicle (i.e. the word or concept used to substitute another word or concept) and the target (i.e. the replaced word or concept), which come from the same conceptual domain. From the perspective of the function of metonymy, Croft (1993, 2002) argues that metonymy highlights one domain within a concept's domain matrix. In a metonymic expression, the concept that a lexical choice represents lies in a domain which belongs to a bigger and more complicated domain matrix. The domain highlighted by the lexical choice can be used to represent another domain in the domain matrix or represent the entire domain matrix.

From the view of profile, Croft and Cruse (2004) define metonymy as an ability of a speaker to select a different contextually salient concept profile in a domain or domain matrix than the one usually symbolized by the word, who divide cognitive construal into four categories; among these categories, metonymy can be realized by the selection operation which falls in the attention/salient category. In other words, the selected concept is profiled to become the figure or focus in one's mental representation of metonymy whilst other parts only become the ground which provides a reference frame to characterize the figure (Talmy 2000). Metonymy here is explained from the perspective of cognitive construal.

Radden and Kövecses (1999: 21) suggest that metonymy is a cognitive process in which the vehicle provides a mental assessment to the target, within the same domain, or ICM initiated by Lakoff (1987). The notion of ICM provides enormous explanatory power to metonymy and is mentioned while defining the metonymy. Inspired by Lakoff (1987), Croft and Cruse (2004) define ICM as a frame presenting an idealized version of the world that simply does not include all possible real-world situations. From Croft and Cruse's (2004) definition, we may discover that ICM is a highly abstract and conceptualized model which usually does not represent reality. For instance, the ICM of BREAKFAST can be portrayed as: MORNING, AFTER SLEEPING, FOOD etc. (Croft & Cruse 2004). The description of the entity and characteristics in an ICM is a complex and boundless gestalt which represents a completed structure, containing many cognitive models. Drawing insights from the notion of ICM, Kövecses and Radden (1998) argue that the mental process of metonymy takes place within the same ICM. Two sub-types of the selection of vehicle and target are identified: between the entire ICM and part of an ICM, or between two parts of an ICM.

The overall evolution of research on metonymy follows a pattern containing four phases: studies on its nature, taxonomy and operating model (Ullmann 1962; Lakoff & Johnson 1980, 1999; Radden & Kövecses 1999); research on metonymy applied in different linguistic levels; studies on the relationship between metonymy and metaphor; and cross-disciplinary studies of metonymy and other theories, such as the critical metonymy analyses aforementioned. Currently, the third and fourth phases still need constant progress and need to be further constructed and completed (Barnden 2010; H. Zhang & T. W. Zhang 2012).

To sum up, the cognitive point of view tends to regard metonymy as a cognitive process or operation which involves the highlighting of one concept or domain in order to represent or provide assessments to another concept or domain. Both concepts and domains should fall within the same domain or domain matrix, echoing with the notion of contiguity.

4.3.2 Classification of metonymy

Cognitive linguistics sheds light on the research of metonymy, providing a new perspective for classifying metonymy. However, in contrast to the classification of metaphor, the cognitive classifying method of metonymy is less standardized. Cognitive linguists classify metonymy from different perspectives, providing different ways of classifying metonymy. Echoing with the rhetoric view of metonymy, the traditional classifying methods are rhetoric in nature. Ullmann (1962) classifies metonymy into three different categories, namely A WHOLE AND ITS PART, AN ACTIVITY AND RELATED PHENOMENA and KINSHIP RELATIONS. However, the major problem with such a classifying method is that it can hardly cover all kinds of metonymic expressions. For example, certain grammatical categories are metonymic in nature. This is the case for the sentence "Mary speaks Chinese". In this sentence, what the speaker actually refers to is that Mary uses Chinese to communicate with people, suggesting certain habitual behaviours or facts by using the present tense to describe the "speaking". This can be treated as a metonymy in which a present event metonymically stands for a habitual event (Wen 2014). However, such metonymic expression does not fall into any of the three categories in Ullmann's (1962) classification. Therefore, his classification lacks explanatory power to some extent. Later, Ungerer and Schmid (2006: 116) propose another classifying method from the perspective of rhetoric, listing nine types of metonymy: (i) part for whole, (ii) whole for part, (iii) container for contents, (iv) material for objects, (v) producer for products, (vi) place for institutions, (vii) place for events, (viii) controlled for controllers, and (ix) cause for effects. The same problem exists since it cannot cover all situations of using metonymy and standardize the classifying method because the nature of metonymy is not just a figure of speech but also a cognitive tool. Panther and Thornburg (1998, 1999) attempt to classify metonymy based on the pragmatic function of metonymy. Based on Panther and Thornburg's (1999: 335) advice on metonymy classification, the author summarizes their ideals in Figure 4-1.

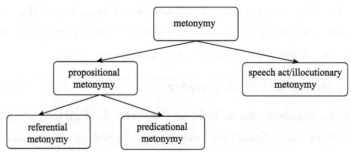

Figure 4-1　Metonymy classification
Note: Summarized from Panther and Thornburg (1999: 335).

Three types of metonymies can be identified in Figure 4-1: referential metonymy, predicational metonymy and speech act/ illocutionary metonymy. Examples of each kind can be illustrated below.

(1) <u>Mozart</u> is on the shelf.

(2) I <u>had to</u> go home.

(3) Can you <u>pass</u> me the salt?

Firstly, referential metonymy stands for the metonymy which is closely related to referencing one entity or concept with another. In sentence (1), "Mozart" is used to refer to the work of Mozart like a music score. Secondly, predicational metonymy employs one expression to refer to a different one. In sentence (2), "I had to go home" stands for a requirement literally, but it metonymically refers to a different statement "I have already homed", which suggests a fact. Lastly, speech act or illocutionary metonymy represents one kind of entity or concept in a speech act standing for another one. In sentence (3), the illocutionary meaning of the sentence is to require the hearer to pass the salt to the speaker. This should be the intended meaning of the speaker, instead of the literal meaning of questioning the hearer's ability to pass salt, which would be quite abnormal in most circumstances. One problem with their classifying method is that their classification only examines the metonymy from the perspective of pragmatics, ignoring the functioning mechanism and cognitive process of metonymy.

Seto (1999: 98) classifies metonymy based on the characteristics of contiguity a metonymy has. The classification can be represented in Figure 4-2.

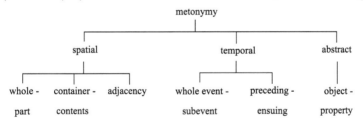

Figure 4-2   Seto's metonymy classification (Seto 1999: 98)

Note: spatial means spatial metonymy; temporal means temporal metonymy; abstract means abstract metonymy; whole–part means whole for part metonymy; container–contents means container for contents metonymy; adjacency means adjacency metonymy; whole event–subevent means whole event for subevent metonymy; preceding–ensuing means preceding for ensuing metonymy; object–property means object for property metonymy.

In Figure 4-2, metonymy is initially divided into three categories, i.e. spatial metonymy, temporal metonymy and abstract metonymy. Seto's classification gives full consideration to the relationship between the metonymy and the world. Then, six sub-types of metonymy are listed. Here, the author takes three of them, namely whole for part metonymy, whole event for subevent metonymy, and object for property metonymy as examples to illustrate such a classifying method.

> (4) I live in the Maple Street.
> (5) Tom went to the cinema.
> (6) This seat is reserved for the old.

In sentence (4), "the Maple Street" is a larger concept, with houses and buildings in it. "The Maple Street" here metonymically stands for a house in the Maple Street where the speaker lives, which shows spatial contiguity in this metonymic expression. Sentence (5) indicates that Tom went out and saw a movie in the cinema. This is an abstract event which consists of many subevents including "leave home", "buy a ticket", "enter the movie hall", "watch the movie", etc. However, the speaker only uses one subevent, i.e. "went to the cinema" to metaphorically refer to the whole event, which exemplifies the "subevent for whole event" metonymy. Sentence (6) contains a metonymic expression of "object/property", with "old" standing for the aged people since old is a major property that aged people have. This classification attempts to sort the metonymy based on the domain to which the contiguity of a metonymy belongs, which greatly contributes to the cognitive study of metonymy. However, classifying methods of metonymy with better systematicness and comprehensiveness is still required considering the complexity of metonymy applications in contexts.

Based on the previous studies, Peirsman and Geeraerts (2006) provide a new classification, summarizing twenty-three types of general metonymy. Thorough as they are, simply listing twenty-three categories of metonymy may seem rather confusing since each category is named by its source. Therefore, these general metonymy types are further grouped into four broader categories based on the domain to which the contiguity of a metonymy belongs (Peirsman & Geeraerts 2006). The four categories will be addressed respectively below.

The first category refers to contiguity in the spatial and material domain. Peirsman and Geeraerts (2006: 279) suggest that six categories of metonymy belong to this kind of contiguity, namely SPATIAL PART FOR WHOLE & WHOLE FOR SPATIAL PART metonymy, LOCATION & LOCATED metonymy, CONTAINER & CONTAINED metonymy, MATERIAL & OBJECT metonymy, PIECE OF CLOTHING & PERSON metonymy, PIECE OF CLOTHING & BODY PART metonymy. Here, the author provides an example of SPATIAL PART & WHOLE metonymy.

(7) Tina will go to <u>America</u> next week.

Here, "America" stands for "the United States of America". Sentence (7) suggests that Tina's destination is a country, i.e. the U.S. However, the entire continent of America is metonymically mentioned here, which falls into the WHOLE FOR SPATIAL PART metonymy.

The second one refers to contiguity in the temporal domain. Three categories are TEMPORAL PART & WHOLE metonymy, ANTECEDENT & CONSEQUENT metonymy, TIME & ENTITY metonymy (Peirsman & Geeraerts 2006). Among them, Peirsman and Geeraerts (2006) argue that the TIME & ENTITY metonymy is incorporated with the metaphor "TIME IS A CONTAINER". Evidence can be seen in Sentence (8).

(8) <u>9-11</u> will never be forgotten. (Peirsman & Geeraerts 2006: 288)

In Sentence (8), "9-11" means September 11th in this sentence, a date which will be long remembered by every American. In this sentence, the date is metaphorically regarded as a container, containing many events inside. Here, "9-11" metonymically refers to an incident taking place on that day.

The third category refers to contiguity in actions, events and processes, including SUBEVENT & COMPLEX EVENT metonymy, ACTION/EVENT/ PROCESS & STATE metonymy, ACTION/EVENT/PROCESS & PARTICIPANT metonymy, CAUSE & EFFECT metonymy (including EFFECT FOR CAUSE metonymy), and PARTICIPANT & PARTICIPANT metonymy. According to Peirsman and Geeraerts (2006), the actions, events and processes domain of contiguity combines both spatial and temporal contiguity together since there are not only temporal entities but also spatial participants in any action, event or process. Taking the CAUSE & EFFECT metonymy as an example, we find that both cause and effect are components of one action, event or process while they are sharing a relationship of sequential order in the time line. Sentence (9) contains a metonymy of such kind.

(9) He was a failure.

In Sentence (9), "failure" is an effect of certain causes; there must be reasons for calling anyone a failure. But in Sentence (9), "a failure" stands for many possible aspects in which "he" fails, what are the causes for calling him "a failure", the effects. Therefore, this sentence contains an EFFECT FOR CAUSE metonymy.

The last contiguity category refers to contiguity in assemblies and collections, including CHARACTERISTIC & ENTITY metonymy, INDIVIDUAL & COLLECTION metonymy, OBJECT & QUANTITY metonymy, CENTRAL FACTOR & INSTITUTION metonymy, HYPONYM & HYPERONYM metonymy (Peirsman & Geeraerts 2006: 301). Sentence (6) which is employed to explain Seto's (1999) classification antecedently, is a good example of the CHARACTERISTIC & ENTITY metonymy.

According to Zhang and Lu (2010), Peirsman and Geeraerts' classification views metonymy as a prototypically structured category, classifying metonymy into different categories based on the contiguous relationship, which are then further sorted based on their domain, strength of contact and boundedness. Thus, having considered the above classifications, the author lists a more comprehensive one in Figure 4-3.

This classifying method provides a comprehensive analysis and explanation cognitively. In particular, the events, actions and processes category focuses on the metonymic relation in an event, action or process, which is also one of the anchor points of this chapter, which analyses metonymy by using the Event-domain Cognitive Model (ECM) theory. Therefore, Peirsman and Geeraerts's (2006) classification of metonymy will be adopted as the standard for classifying metonymy in this research.

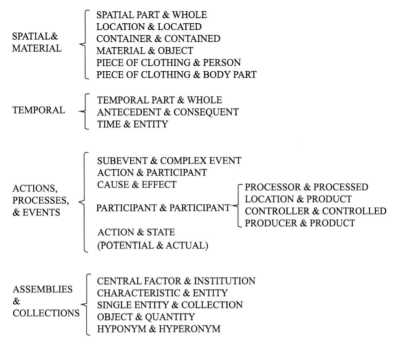

Figure 4-3 A comprehensive classification of metonymy

Note: The word "metonymy" at the end of all metonymy types is omitted.

4.4 Metonymy Identification and Classification from the Data

Radden and Kövecses (1999) argue that conceptual relationships within an ICM that generate metonymies are called "metonymy-producing relationships" and people's knowledge about the world is organized by structured ICMs which people perceive as wholes with parts. The author will use the term metonymy types to replace metonymy–producing relationships as Littlemore (2015) does. In Table 4-2, the author summarizes ICM types and their taxonomy based on Radden and Kövecses's (1999, 2007) studies.

Table 4-2 ICM types and their taxonomy

Whole ICM and its part(s)	Examples	Parts of an ICM	Examples
thing and part ICM	whole for a part: America for the United States of America part of whole: London for England	action ICM	They summered at Ville d'Vvary.

continued

Whole ICM and its part(s)	Examples	Parts of an ICM	Examples
scale ICM	whole for upper end: You are speeding again. upper end for the whole: How old are you?	perception ICM	a gorgeous sight
constitution ICM	object for material: I smell skunk. material for object: wood for "forest"	causation ICM	You are a success.
event ICM	whole for sub: Bill smoked marijuana. sub for whole: Mary speaks Spanish.	production ICM	He drives a Ford.
category and member ICM	category for a member: He comes around for some drinks. member for category: aspirin for any pain-reliving tablets	control ICM	Mrs. Grundy frowns on blue jeans.
category and property ICM	category for salient: brain for "intelligence" salient for category: Blacks for "black people"	possession ICM	He married money.
reduction ICM	part of a form for the whole: crude for crude oil	containment ICM	The bottle is sour.
—	—	location ICM	The whole town showed up.
—	—	sign and reference ICM	a self-contradictory utterance
—	—	modification ICM	LOL

In Table 4-2, there are seven ICMs in the category of whole ICM and its part(s), and ten types are included in the category of parts of an ICM. Each ICM is explained with an example. Based on the source and target of the metonymy, the author highlights different types of metonymies in discourses, discussing the cognitive process in decoding them and revealing underlying cognitive and cultural implications.

In total, 474 types of metonymy are identified, with 251 in English texts and 223 in Chinese texts. On the ground of Peirsman and Geeraerts's (2006) classification of metonymy, thirteen metonymy types appear in English texts and fourteen in Chinese texts; the top five and their frequencies and percentages are displayed in Table 4-3.

Table 4-3 Metonymy in English and Chinese texts

Metonymy type	Metonymy in English texts		Metonymy in Chinese texts	
	Frequency	Percentage	Frequency	Percentage
CAUSE & EFFECT	78	**31.08%**	72	**32.29%**
SUBEVENT & COMPLEX EVENT	43	17.13%	62	**27.80%**
COLLECTION & SINGLE ENTITY	53	**21.12%**	17	7.62%
ENTITY & CHARACTERISTIC	27	10.76%	21	9.42%
ACTION & STATE	15	5.98%	23	10.31%
Other metonymy types in total	35	13.93%	28	12.56%
Total	251	100.00%	223	100.00%

This section only analyse the four most frequent metonymy types in each corpus. The author will analyse four typologies of metonymy in PoV. CAUSE & EFFECT metonymy occurs most frequently in both Chinese and English texts, whilst there are linguistic differences regarding metonymic uses in both texts. For instance, except for CAUSE & EFFECT metonymy, English writers prefer to use COLLECTION & SINGLE ENTITY metonymy in PoV more, followed by SUBEVENT & COMPLEX EVENT. As for Chinese texts, the second preferred type of metonymy is SUBEVENT & COMPLEX EVENT, while the third preferred type is ACTION & STATE. Their detailed linguistic variations of PoV will be analysed in section 4.5.

4.5 Metonymic PoV Grammar in Promotional Discourses of Anti-Cancer Medicines

Having identified the metonymies applied in both Chinese and English data, the author analyses their applications in PoV structure to illustrate their meanings in discourses, so as to reveal different assumptions of cognitive views in different contexts and different cultures. Meanwhile, the foci of cognitive selection of metonymic PoV in promotional discourses displays the cognitive preferences of institutional discourse patterns in different cultures as well.

4.5.1 $X_2Y_4Z_4$ and $X_2Y_4Z_3$ viewpoints

$X_2Y_4Z_4$ and $X_2Y_4Z_3$ points of view share certain commonalities as they both represent an observing point with a left side anchor and bird's eyes angle. The minor differences lie in the appearance of previous events and causations. Nevertheless, they share similar implications in terms of the interpretations of the PoV, and therefore can be together analysed.

$X_2Y_4Z_4$ and $X_2Y_4Z_3$ represent viewpoints which are formed by a left side anchor, a bird's eye angle and a medium or long shot distance. Such viewpoints are largely employed to construct sentences containing metonymic types like ENTITY FOR CHARACTERISTIC, COLLECTION FOR SINGLE ENTITY, EFFECT FOR CAUSE, COMPLEX EVENT FOR SYBEVENT, etc.

From the $X_2Y_4Z_4$ point of view, three elements can be identified. First, X_2 represents a left side anchor, which, according to Hart (2015), invites the reader to "take sides". That is, readers do not observe the actions and entities from an unbiased anchor point; instead, they are sharing the same viewpoint with the agent of the sentence. X_2 anchor is generally realized by the active sentence in which the agent(s) of an asymmetrical action is/are primarily introduced to the reader. Second, Y_4 stands for the angle of the bird's eyes. That happens when one looks down from the top; we might have similar experiences when we stand on a building and look down to the floor. Y_4 generally appears in a sentence with a loss in granularity, which means that individual elements in the semantic construction are hard to be identified; they are replaced by a description of the rough outline of an event, process or action, which generally closely relates to some nominalized expressions and whole for part metonymies (Talmy 2000; Hart 2015). It displays a bigger picture of the described event, process or action, ignoring some details therein. Third, Z_4 long shot distance can be found in a sentence which includes not only the agent and patient of a sentence, but also the causational clauses that express previous events or actions closely related to the main clause, expressing causation or time. Therefore, Z_4 provides more information in a sentence and enlarges the viewing frame of the reader. The only difference between $X_2Y_4Z_4$ and $X_2Y_4Z_3$ PoVs lies in the distance point. Z_3 distance point, as explained earlier, contains a smaller viewing frame than that of Z_4. Therefore, the linguistic representation with a Z_4 distance point only contains the agent and patient, omitting any causational clause.

In the Anti-Cancer medicine promotional discourses, examples of the $X_2Y_4Z_4$ and $X_2Y_4Z_3$ viewpoints can be well illustrated in the following sentences.

Example 1 (Source: ET2)

Patients in the U.S. have access to Pfizer Oncology Together™, which offers personalized support and financial assistance resources to help patients access their prescribed Pfizer Oncology medications. (U.S. FDA Approves DAURISMO™ (glasdegib) for Adult Patients with Newly-Diagnosed Acute Myeloid Leukemia (AML) for Whom Intensive Chemotherapy Is Not an Option, Pfizer, 21 November, 2018)[1]

Example 2 (Source: ET2)

Historically, a majority of these individuals do not receive treatment and face a poor prognosis. (U.S. FDA Approves DAURISMO™ (glasdegib) for Adult Patients with Newly-Diagnosed Acute Myeloid Leukemia (AML) for Whom Intensive Chemotherapy is Not an Option, Pfizer, 21 November, 2018)[2]

Example 3 (Source: ET29)

Eli Lilly and Company (NYSE: LLY) today announced that Verzenio (abemaciclib) demonstrated a statistically significant improvement in overall survival in the Phase 3 MONARCH 2 clinical trial. (Lilly's Verzenio® (abemaciclib) Significantly Extended Life in Women with HR+, HER2- Advanced Breast Cancer in MONARCH 2, Lilly, 30 July, 2019)[3]

Example 4 (Source: CT8)

中山大学肿瘤防治中心张力教授团队研究证实，国产 PD-1 免疫治疗

---

[1] https://www.pfizer.com/news/press-release/press-release-detail/u_s_fda_approves_daurismo_glasdegib_for_adult_patients_with_newly_diagnosed_acute_myeloid_leukemia_aml_for_whom_intensive_chemotherapy_is_not_an_option

[2] https://www.pfizer.com/news/press-release/press-release-detail/u_s_fda_approves_daurismo_glasdegib_for_adult_patients_with_newly_diagnosed_acute_myeloid_leukemia_aml_for_whom_intensive_chemotherapy_is_not_an_option

[3] https://investor.lilly.com/news-releases/news-release-details/lillys-verzenior-abemaciclib-significantly-extended-life-women

药物卡瑞利珠单抗对复发转移的鼻咽癌疗效显著。(鼻咽癌治疗获新突破 国产 PD-1 治疗鼻咽癌将给患者带来福音，恒瑞医药/新华网，2018 年 9 月 29 日)[①]

The research conducted by Professor Zhang's team from Sun Yat-Sen University Cancer Centre (SYSUCC) has confirmed that domestic PD-1 immunotherapy medicine Camrelizumab has prominent curative effects on the recurrence and metastasis of nasopharyngeal cancer. (New breakthrough in nasopharyngeal cancer treatment: domestic PD-1 treatment of nasopharyngeal cancer brings good news to patients, Hengrui Pharma /Xinhua Net, 29 September, 2018)

Example 5 (Source: CT8)

国产药物的价格一定会优于进口药，在医保谈判时能显出优势，可尽快纳入医保。(鼻咽癌治疗获新突破 国产 PD-1 治疗鼻咽癌将给患者带来福音，恒瑞医药/新华网，2018 年 9 月 29 日)[②]

The price of domestic drugs definitely precedes that of imported drugs, which shows an advantage in the health insurance negotiation and can be included in the health insurance in a short time. (New breakthrough in nasopharyngeal cancer treatment: domestic PD-1 treatment of nasopharyngeal cancer brings good news to patients, Hengrui Pharma/ Xinhua Net, 29 September, 2018)

In Example 1, Pfizer, the company, is the agent of the action offering support and assistance to patients. The readers (might be doctors, patients and their relatives), who have taken the same viewing side as the agent, would be more likely to comprehend and agree with the company's action of bringing benefits to the patients. The phrases "personalized support" and "financial assistance" contain two COLLECTION FOR SINGLE ENTITY metonymies, which are constructed through two nominal "support" and "assistance", which contain multiple components semantically. Ignoring the single entity and applying a collection item can provide a bigger picture to readers, making them understand what the "help" means to the patients in general, and building up a responsible and reliable image of the company. A causational clause suggesting

---

① http://m.xinhuanet.com/health/2018-09/29/c_1123504909.htm
② http://m.xinhuanet.com/health/2018-09/29/c_1123504909.htm

the accessibility of Pfizer underpins such an image and further promotes this company. In Example 2, "a majority of these individuals... face a poor prognosis" suggests that the lack of treatment methods is a serious problem, emphasizing the great necessity and significance of the new medicine DAURISMO. Similarly, the readers may find it easier to accept this opinion since they take the agent's view, i.e. the cancer patient's side, which may lead them to feel nervous, and who may attach more importance to this issue. An EVENT FOR SUBEVENT metonymy "face a poor prognosis", which comprises several events like facing negative outcomes, losing faith and getting worse, provides the readers with mental assessments to the issue of how bad AML patients can get without proper drug therapy. In combination with the semantic implication of metonymy, such a grammatical construction emphasizes the great necessity and significance of the new medicine DAURISMO, and therefore helps promote this new medicine to AML patients. Example 3 states that Verzenio has a "statistically significant improvement in overall survival", which is the result of Verzenio exterminating the cancer cell and curing the disease. Here, the trial result is perceived as a thing or a whole. The discourse producer briefly describes the trial result as an improvement so that the reader can instantly understand the superiority of the medicine.

The same viewpoint can also be identified when the Chinese texts are examined. In Example 4, Camrelizumab has "prominent curative effects" on the nasopharyngeal cancer. When patients with this type of cancer read this report, they may conceptualize this medicine as a fighter just like them, who actively fight against the cancer and strive for victory. The EFFECT FOR CAUSE metonymy "疗效显著", i.e. "has prominent curative effects" provides confidence in the medicine to the patient. A previous causational clause also suggests that these effects are proved and justified by a research conducted by a team of outstanding experts who have worked in this field for years, which adds reliability to the information. In Example 5, "shows an advantage" is also an EFFECT FOR CAUSE metonymy, which also hints about the good quality and low price of the new medicine. The writer also invites the readers to observe the action of "precede" from the agent's viewpoint, i.e. the new medicine's viewpoint, which builds up a similar cognition related to the advantages of the new medicine in the reader's mind so as to promote the new

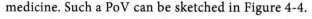

medicine. Such a PoV can be sketched in Figure 4-4.

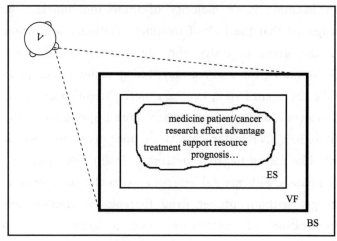

Figure 4-4 $X_2Y_4Z_4$ and $X_2Y_4Z_3$ viewpoints in Anti-Cancer medicine promotion
Note: In figures throughout this book, V means viewer.

In Figure 4-4, an $X_2Y_4Z_4$ and $X_2Y_4Z_3$ viewpoints show that the writer wants to guide his readers to perceive the medicine or the corporation itself from the agent's perspective; in other words, the writer wants readers to be actively involved in the discourse, sharing the same perspective with him/her. Meanwhile, the writer also wants to lead readers to a higher position with a long or relatively long distance so that readers are able to get a bigger picture instead of scrutinizing the components, detailed causes and characteristics. By doing so, on the one hand, the information is easier to be accepted by the readers since they share the same viewing direction with the agent, which is generally the medicine, or the company that has developed it; on the other hand, collective and general descriptions of the individual elements allow the readers to receive a general understanding of the issues addressed, which facilitates them to build up a clearer cognition about the issue, leaving a deeper impression of the promoted medicine in their minds. The impression will also be stressed if previous causational and temporal clauses exist, because readers, such as patients with little knowledge about Anti-Cancer medicine will gain a better understanding concerning a specific type of medicine, forming an overall favourable impression to the medicine or even to the entire company in their mind, which makes them be more willing to choose the medicine when they are in need. Meanwhile, if a doctor who finds a proper medicine to treat his/her patient, he/she may try this new medicine if the same impression has been formed in his or her mind. In aggregation, the promotional effect of the discourse has been well achieved.

4.5.2　$X_4Y_2Z_4$ and $X_4Y_2Z_3$ viewpoints

$X_4Y_2Z_4$ **and** $X_4Y_2Z_3$ points of view contain a right side anchor, a default sightline and a long shot distance. While the medium and long shot distance has been explained above, the explanations to the other two variables are necessary. A right side anchor implies that the viewer shares the same viewpoint with the patient of the sentence to observe the scene whilst a default sightline suggests that the viewer places himself in the same horizontal plane with the scene, observing it equally, which makes the detail, component and process more visible in the following examples.

> **Example 6 (Source: ET24)**
>
> ... in patients who received VENCLYXTO plus rituximab, resulting in an 83 percent reduction in the risk of disease progression or death (hazard ratio [HR]:0.17; 95% confidence interval [CI]: 0.11-0.25; P<0.0001)... (AbbVie Receives European Commission Approval of VENCLYXTO® (venetoclax) Plus Rituximab for the Treatment of Patients with Chronic Lymphocytic Leukemia Who Have Received at Least One Prior Therapy, Abbvie, 1 November, 2018)[1]
>
> **Example 7 (Source: ET20)**
>
> With the approval of this new indication, patients in Japan with BRCA-mutated advanced ovarian cancer who respond to chemotherapy will have the opportunity to benefit from LYNPARZA in the first-line maintenance setting. (AstraZeneca and Merck's LYNPARZA® (olaparib) Approved in Japan as First-Line Maintenance Therapy in Patients with BRCA-Mutated Advanced Ovarian Cancer, Merck, 19 June, 2019)[2]

[1] https://news.abbvie.com/news/press-releases/abbvie-receives-european-commission-approval-venclyxto-venetoclax-plus-rituximab-for-treatment-patients-with-chronic-lymphocytic-leukemia-who-have-received-at-least-one-prior-therapy.htm

[2] https://www.merck.com/news/astrazeneca-and-mercks-lynparza-olaparib-approved-in-japan-as-first-line-maintenance-therapy-in-patients-with-brca-mutated-advanced-ovarian-cancer/

Example 8 (Source: CT9)

结果显示，单药治疗组，有 34%的患者肿瘤体积缩小超过 50%，总计 59%的患者肿瘤**得到了控制**，中位无疾病进展时间达到了 5.6 个月。(鼻咽癌治疗获新突破 国产 PD-1 治疗鼻咽癌将给患者带来福音，恒瑞医药/新华网，2018 年 9 月 29 日)[①]

Results showed that 34% of patients in the monotherapy group had tumours that shrank by more than 50%, a total of 59% **had tumours under control**, and the median disease-free time was 5.6 months. (New breakthrough in nasopharyngeal cancer treatment: domestic PD-1 treatment of nasopharyngeal cancer brings good news to patients, Hengrui Pharma/Xinhuanet, 29 September, 2018)

Example 9 (Source: CT9)

在肿瘤免疫治疗**大热**的当下，PD-1 免疫检查点抑制剂在鼻咽癌领域**取得了突破**，给患者带来长期生存的希望。(鼻咽癌治疗获新突破 国产 PD-1 治疗鼻咽癌将给患者带来福音，恒瑞医药/新华网，2018 年 9 月 29 日)[②]

Under **the currently hot trend** of tumour immunotherapy, PD-1 immuno checkpoint inhibitors have **made a breakthrough** in the field of nasopharyngeal cancer, bringing hopes of long-term survival to patients. (New breakthrough in nasopharyngeal cancer treatment: domestic PD-1 treatment of nasopharyngeal cancer brings good news to patients, Hengrui Pharma/Xinhuanet, 29 September, 2018)

In the above excerpts, the anchor point gradually shifts to that of the cancer patients. The discourse producers adopt such a point of view that the reader perceives himself as a cancer patient who suffers from the disease and is desperately in need of proper medicines. It positions the readers on the side of the cancer patients so that the discourse readers can easily share their feeling with the patients and understand the situation faced by the patients. The medical process and pain brought by the cancer come directly toward the readers, and solutions have to be found. Meanwhile, a default sightline angle provides a plain viewpoint which allows the reader to observe the individual

---

[①] http://www.shhrp.com/news/group_news/1539571539.html

[②] http://www.shhrp.com/news/group_news/1539571539.html

elements inside including the patient, medicine, treatment, links of the treatment process. Besides, a medium to long distance includes both the patient (cancer patients) and the agent (cancer, medicine, treatment, etc.) of the linguistic representation, making both of them visible to the readers.

In Example 6, the pharmaceutical company Abbvie hopes to justify the treating effect of their medicine VENCLYXTO plus rituximab. The combination of the two medicines is a new attempt, so evidences and proofs for the therapeutic effects must be provided in order to gain credibilities. The discourse producer then provides an intended result which shows that the patients who receive VENCLYXTO plus rituximab are actually 83 percent less likely to have a cancer progression or death. This sentence explicitly indicates the positive effects and outcomes brought to the patients by the new drug combination. The agent of the sentence, i.e. the VENCLYXTO plus rituximab and the cancer patients of the sentence, is explicitly shown in the sentence to deepen the reader's impression, and specific data of the trial result is presented at the end of the sentence to make the result more convincing. Similarly, in Example 7, patients with BRCA-mutated advanced ovarian cancer in Japan are accepting benefits from the LYNPARZA. The previous phrase "With the approval of this new indication" provides the reason why Japanese customers have accessed to the LYNPARZA, that means, the medicine is approved by Japan's Pharmaceuticals and Medical Devices Agency (PMDA), a regulatory agency with a great reputation. It adds even more credibility to LYNPARZA for the fact that PMDA is an authoritative agency in the medical field. Similar to Example 6, Example 9 is subsumed within the EFFECT FOR CAUSE metonymy "取得了突破 made a breakthrough". The effect of PD-1 treatment is employed to construct the cause thereof, which aims at revealing the information that the reader deems crucial: the effect of controlling the tumor by using a concrete percentage of the treatment effect. While in Example 8, instead of describing any specific therapeutic effect, the EFFECT FOR CAUSE metonymy "得到了控制 had... under control" draws the public attention to the popularity and development of the medicines. The PoV cognitive process can be sketched as in Figure 4-5.

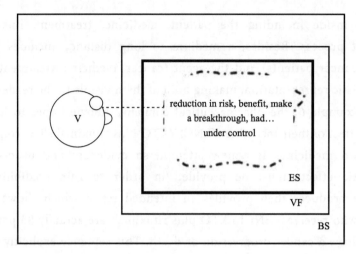

Figure 4-5   X₄Y₂Z₄ and X₄Y₂ Z₃ viewpoints in Anti-Cancer medicine promotion

In Figure 4-5, a PoV of $X_4Y_2Z_4$ or $X_4Y_2Z_3$ takes the patients' side to construct the scene. Readers in this viewpoint perceive themselves as the second patients in the scene, and the action is approaching the patients as well as the readers. The discourse producer wants to put the readers in the patients' shoes so that it may trigger the same feelings or ideas inside the readers' minds. Since the cancer patients generally serve as the patients of the sentence, the readers will generate sympathy for and consonance with them and then realize the importance of the Anti-Cancer medicines. A default sightline angle point in a combination of a medium or long-distance point allows the readers to have a comprehensive view of the scene. On the one hand, the default sightline demonstrates all the elements involved in an action. Under the purpose of making the readers feel for the cancer patients, instead of giving an obscure framework of the described event, the discourse producer needs to provide more details and introduce the individual elements involved in the event, so as to make the statement more convincing and evidential. On the other hand, the medium or long distance helps the readers clearly identify the agents and patients, and clarify the entire process of actions like "cancer patients can obtain benefits from the new medicine" or "cancer patient is tortured by the illness".

As illustrated above, promoting the company's medicine is one of the major functions of the Anti-Cancer medicine promotional discourse. For Anti-Cancer medicine, potential customers generally include cancer patients, doctors and medical researchers. For a cancer patient, if he/she suffers from the same type of cancer as the one described in the discourse, he/she could have the feeling of finding a life saviour as he/she reads the discourse. Similar situations prompt him/her to search for more about the medicine, so as to stimulate the purchasing behaviour eventually. For a medical personnel, the patient's situation and full demonstration of the medicine can in a way arouse people's interest in the medicine, which also encourages the selection of the medicine for either therapeutic purposes or research purposes.

4.5.3 $X_1Y_4Z_3$ viewpoint

The $X_1Y_4Z_3$ viewpoint includes a front side anchor, bird's eye angle and medium distance. Unlike the X_2 or X_4 anchor point which takes the side of either agent or patient, the X_1 anchor point takes the viewer to an unbiased position to observe the described scene. In Anti-Cancer medicine promotional discourses, the $X_1Y_4Z_3$ viewpoint is generally used to compare the medicine with previous medicines or medical indexes. The following examples show how the viewpoint is applied.

> **Example 10 (Source: ET1)**
> This includes results from the phase 3 REFLECTIONS B739-03 clinical comparative study, which demonstrated <u>clinical equivalence</u> and found <u>no clinically meaningful differences</u> between ZIRABEV and Avastin in patients with advanced non-squamous NSCLC. (Pfizer Receives Positive CHMP Opinion for Oncology Biosimilar, ZIRABEV™ (bevacizumab), Pfizer, 14 December, 2018)[1]
>
> **Example 11 (Source: ET14)**
> Long-term safety data for Opdivo from all four studies <u>were consistent with</u> the known adverse event profile and did not reveal any new safety signals. (Bristol-Myers Squibb Announces Long-Term Survival Results from Pooled Analyses of Opdivo (nivolumab) in Previously-Treated Non-Small

---

[1] https://www.pfizer.com/news/press-release/press-release-detail/pfizer_receives_positive_chmp_opinion_for_oncology_ biosimilar_zirabev_bevacizumab

Cell Lung Cancer Patients, Bristol-Myers Squibb, 2 April, 2019)①

Example 12 (Source: CT4)

复星凯特作为中国**第一梯队**的 CAR-T 药品研发企业，借助 KITE PHARMA 先进的 CAR-T 治疗技术、复星深厚的医药健康产业基础和吉利德公司丰富的医药产品商业化经验，定将开创中国细胞免疫治疗产业化发展的新纪元。(复星凯特开启全球首款获批 CAR-T 产品 Yescarta 在中国产业化征程，复星医药，2017 年 12 月 6 日)②

As **a first echelon** CAR-T medicine R&D enterprise in China, FosunKite will create a new era of the industrialization of cellular immunotherapy in China with the help of KITE PHARMA's advanced CAR-T therapy technology, our profound foundation in health industry and Gilead's experience in the commercialization of pharmaceutical products. (FosunKite initiates the industrialization journey of Yescarta, the first globally approved CAR-T product, Fosun Pharma, 6 December, 2017)

Example 13 (Source: CT17)

……在 PD-1 的研发策略上，不但有信心汇聚全国肿瘤界的顶尖专家，聚力前行，更有信心以未来一系列**重拳**举措，通过 GLS-010 有效开拓中国肿瘤免疫市场，为中国患者提供优质、可负担的创新型药物，助力提升大众健康水平。(严控质量，聚力前行：誉衡药业 PD-1 启动关键注册上市研究，誉衡药业，2018 年 6 月 20 日)③

… In terms of the R&D strategy of PD-1, we not only have the confidence of gathering the top experts in the field of oncology in China and forging ahead, but also believe in effectively expanding the Chinese tumour immune market through GLS-010 with **a heavy fist**, so as to provide high-quality and affordable innovative drugs for Chinese patients and to help improve the public health level. (Strict control of quality, combined force and step forward: Yuheng Medicine's PD-1 launched key research of registration and listing, Yuheng Medicine, 20 June, 2018)

Example 10 compares the therapeutic effect between the newly-developed

---

① https://news.bms.com/news/corporate-financial/2019/Bristol-Myers-Squibb-Announces-Long-Term-Survival-Results-from-Pooled-Analyses-of-Opdivo-nivolumab-in-Previously-Treated-Non-Small-Cell-Lung-Cancer-Patients/default.aspx

② https://www.fosunpharma.com/content/details37_7237.html

③ http://www.gloria.cc/index.php?m=content&c=index&a=show&catid=74&id=428

medicine ZIRABEV and the original medicine Avastin. Avastin is an antineoplastic agent invented in 2004. After multiple tests throughout the last decade, it has already become a highly recognized medicine. ZIRABEV, according to the original text, is a potential biosimilar to Avastin. Therefore, whether ZIRABEV can be a qualified alternative for Avastin or not is a major concern of the public. Therefore, to convince the reader, discourse producers lead the readers to the middle point in front of the two agents. With agent one (ZIRABEV) and agent two (Avastin) presented on the left and right side respectively, collective and nominalized terms "clinical equivalence" and "no clinically meaningful difference" are employed to describe their therapeutic effect. Individual causes for "clinical equivalence" like having the same effects, side effects and treatment cycle are omitted from a bird's eye angle, which makes it an EFFECT FOR CAUSE metonymy. Readers, from this point of view, are guided to perceive the ZIRABEV as an acceptable alternative for cancer patients. Similar implications may be identified in Example 11. The comparison is conducted between the safety data of medicine Opdivo and the adverse event profile. Adverse event profile makes the record about adverse response with unascertained causation. For a medicine, being consistent with the adverse event profile means that the property of the medicine remains stable, which is extremely crucial since the medicine is used in a damaged human body, and the medicine itself cannot further exert uncontrollable effects on the body. From the front anchor point, the unbiased position allows the reader to view both the medicine and existing medical index equally, making the first agent match up to the second one.

As for Chinese excerpts, a company's development prospect is supported by the R&D of its products, which attracts potential customers and investors. Here, two commonly used concepts "第一梯队 a first echelon" in Example 12 and "重拳 a heavy fist" in Example 13 serve as sources of metonymy, to construct the target concept, i.e. the strength of the company and the product. In Chinese culture, "a first echelon" represents the elite class relatively, symbolizing the possession of wealth, technology, and skills at the highest level. Meanwhile, "a heavy fist" in Chinese indicates the intensiveness and completeness of an action or a move compared to other less invested business. In the discourse context, the first echelon demonstrates Fuxing's leading position in the Chinese pharmaceutical industry, paralleled to other pharmaceutical companies, whilst "a heavy fist" manifests Yuheng's determination in developing and expanding PD-1, both of which inspire confidence in the company and the credibility of its medicines compared to other medicine producers in China. Based on the above interpretations, the $X_1Y_4Z_3$ viewpoint is sketched as in Figure 4-6.

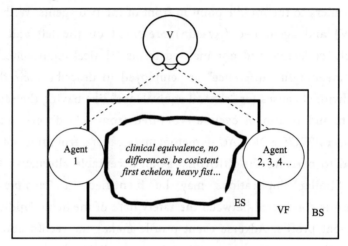

Figure 4-6 $X_1Y_4Z_3$ viewpoint in Anti-Cancer medicine promotion

Overall, in Figure 4-6, one of the most significant characteristics of an $X_1Y_4Z_3$ viewpoint is that it places the readers in the middle of two agents; the readers therefore tend to perceive the two agents in an unbiased manner. When it comes to comparing two medicines or building up a connection between them, especially when a newly-developed medicine is compared to a highly recognized one, the producer needs to persuade the public that the new medicine can reach the standard and perform as well as the original medicine or treatment. Since childhood, human beings have possessed the ability to identify left and right and balance them, and it is their nature that they equally observe their left side and right side. That's why a front anchor makes one treat the agent on the left and right equally. Combined with a medium distance which presents the agent and patient at the same time, and a bird's eye which portrays the general picture of the scene, the front anchor in medicine promotional discourses then invites the readers to actively participate in the process of equalizing the promoted medicine with the original one or medical standard. Together, the discourse producer adopts the $X_1Y_4Z_3$ point of view to guide the potential customer to accept the new medicine so as to achieve better promotion.

4.6 Cross-cultural Differences of Metonymic PoV in Promotional Discourses of Anti-Cancer Medicines

Discourses from different countries and written in different languages embody significant cultural differences. By analysing the metonymy in Sino-American Anti-Cancer medicine promotional discourses, the author decodes the cognitive process beneath metonymic expressions therein to shed light on the promotion strategies and cultural implications embodied in the promotional discourses of Anti-Cancer medicine.

Drawing insights from initial studies, the author identifies that the types of metonymy and the adopted point of view are generally the same in both Chinese and English discourses. However, some similarities and disparities identified in the two kinds of discourses reveal the frequencies of the metonymy types, and the $X_2Y_4Z_4$ viewpoint is employed more in the Chinese discourses than in English discourses. Besides, the same metonymy tends to be used differently in Chinese and English discourses. The author's findings are as follows: (i) Cancer patients, doctors and researchers all over the world may face the same problems and share the same needs as cancer has been a universal challenge to the entire world, which results in similar linguistic strategies like employing such metonymic expressions as CAUSE AND EFFECT, SUBEVENT AND COMPLEX EVENT, ACTION AND STATE, ENTITY AND CHARACTERISTIC, etc. to cater to the needs of the doctors, patients and patient's family members who mainly compose the discourse readers. (ii) Influenced by the enormous cultural differences between China and the U.S., Chinese and American people generally possess an entirely different set of values, norms and social customs. Chinese people tend to believe in authority more and value the reputation and fame of medicine producers whilst American people tend to believe in statistics and facts more, which generates tendencies to select different metonymy types and points of view in Anti-Cancer medicine promotional discourses. (iii) Differences between Chinese and English in linguistic aspects create preferences to certain metonymy types and points of view, like the use of CAUSE AND EFFECT metonymy and active/passive voice. Nevertheless, different applications of metonymy implied diverse interpretations of Anti-Cancer medicine or cancer treatment concerning PoV. The frequency of each metonymy type is shown in Figure 4-7.

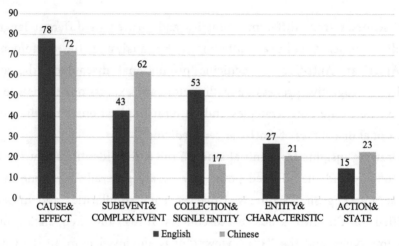

Figure 4-7   Comparison of metonymy types in English and Chinese discourses

Regarding the metonymy types applied in PoV, the combining patterns of points of view can be various and complex in the light of Figures 2-1, 2-2, 2-3 and 2-4. Among all the other frequently used points of views, the $X_2Y_4Z_4$ viewpoint achieves specific cognitive effects of earning the readers' approval more easily, presenting a broad picture of the described event/action/process to the readers and allowing them to receive a general understanding of the current event/action/process and its causation or temporal relations. As has been proven, different points of view may achieve different cognitive effects, which are closely related to certain types of metonymy. Although the $X_2Y_4Z_4$ and $X_2Y_4Z_3$ viewpoints appear in both Chinese and English discourses at a high ratio, the respective frequencies of other viewpoints are different (Table 4-4).

Table 4-4　PoV Occurrences in Medicine Promotional Discourses

Types of PoV	Percentage of CTs	Percentage of ETs
$X_2Y_4Z_4$ / $X_2Y_4Z_3$	34%	36%
$X_4Y_2Z_4$ / $X_4Y_2Z_3$	22%	48%
$X_1Y_4Z_3$	44%	16%
Total	100%	100%

Although the combining patterns of PoV are dynamic and complex, the highly occurred PoVs are $X_2Y_4Z_4$ and $X_2Y_4Z_3$ (a right side anchor, bird's eye angle and a long shot distance), $X_4Y_2Z_4$ and $X_4Y_2Z_3$ (a right side anchor, a default sightline and a long shot distance) and $X_1Y_4Z_3$ (a front side anchor, bird's eye angle and medium distance). Having studied their frequency, the author finds that $X_1Y_4Z_3$ viewpoint appears more in the Chinese discourse, and applies more subjective and comparative metonymies to express the feasibility and validity of the medicines, followed by direct quotations and claims raised by institutions or experts. $X_1Y_4Z_3$ viewpoint related to facts and statistics are also applied and favoured by Chinese discourse writers at the first place, while favoured by English discourse writers at the third place, who pay more attention to the real results of treatment with numbers and percentages. The second preferred viewpoint for English discourse writers is $X_2Y_4Z_4$ / $X_2Y_4Z_3$, showing similar comprehension of and faithfulness to the information and its source coming from pharmaceutical institutions and medical experts. It should be noted that $X_4Y_2Z_4$ and $X_4Y_2Z_3$ viewpoints are least preferred by Chinese discourse writers, who may regard the medicines produced as an individual case, rather than a comparison or competition with others. Such a viewpoint in discourses is more neutral and objective. The cross-cultural differences strongly support that there are preferences concerning the use of grammatical constructions to describe certain metonymic meanings in Chinese and English Anti-Cancer medicine promotional discourses.

The cognition and recognition of linguistic acts require communicators' cultural background and learning experience, their conceptual systems and grammar structure encoded in languages. Under WG, PoV functions within cognitive models where metonymies play roles mainly as CAUSE & EFFECT, SUBEVENT & COMPLEX EVENT, COLLECTION & SINGLE ENTITY,

ENTITY & CHARATERISTIC and ACTION & STATE, referring to various cognitive processes and combining patterns and implicating mental assessments.

4.7   Summary

Cultural differences in discourses concerning cognitive grammar should be considered when an institution wants to promote its products to other cultures. As Yang (2020: 194) suggests, embodied cognitive actions and models exist in different languages of different cultures. Although certain metonymy types and points of view may achieve additional promotion effects, the author argues that discourse producers should be more cautious while using metonymies and points of view in Anti-Cancer medicine promotional discourses. When discourse producers build up a positive image of a kind of medicine, they could potentially prevent patients from choosing the most suitable medicine for patients' lack of relevant knowledge, disallowing them to receive more information related to some negative factors like the side effects, etc. For medical staff and researchers, as potential readers with completely different needs, some subjective evaluative terms, emotional descriptions and obscurities of certain semantic parts may distract them away from unbiased comprehension of medicines, which is crucial for curative and inquisitive purposes for promotion and sales. Therefore, discourse producers must consider the preciseness and completeness of information instead of the pure pursuit of promotion effects, for the reason that the Anti-Cancer medicine promotional discourse integrates the characteristics of both business discourses and medical discourses.

Chapter 5

Force Dynamics in Promotional Discourses of Online Treatments

After the rise of the Internet medical industry, many experts have carried out a variety of application studies on it, such as policy, management and institution. Online medical consultation, as one of the most important new medical industries, is just the tip of the iceberg in the vast business of Internet medical. The emergence and expansion of Internet medical in China is an inevitable event. One of the conditions is the penetration of Internet, the other is the increasing demand of people for medical services, while the medical resources in China are insufficient and unequally distributed. Thus, the appearance of Internet medical alleviates some problems for patients, such as registration difficulty. The release of medical information by professional medical and health service platforms, though not as authoritative as hospitals, is more convenient, quick and easy to obtain for ordinary people. All these are conducive to the development of China's medical industry and the overall improvement of national health. And the application of Internet in medical treatment will develop rapidly in the future, and Internet medical counselling is bound to become an essential part of people's lives, which has been confirmed in recent years, especially after the outbreak of the epidemic in 2020.

5.1　Introduction

Taking the various obstacles existing in the Internet medical industry as the starting point, Li and Sun (2016) conduct an innovative study on it. For example, formulating industry standards and norms, improving the application modes of Internet technology, training general practitioners and other development programs, with a view of promoting better development of Internet medical care. In addition to analysing the pattern and current status of online healthcare, some scholars delve into the impact of "Internet + healthcare" on the traditional medical service mode and the physician-patient relationship. Wang and Feng (2017) argue that "Internet + healthcare" could break down the barriers of information asymmetry between physicians and patients, and could promote the transformation of the medical service mode from "physician-led" to "patient-centred". However, some strategies need to be adopted to deal with the challenges that may arise in the development of online healthcare. This chapter analyses the promotional discourses of online healthcare services from WG perspective by empathizing with the word uses of force dynamics.

5.2　Data for Force Dynamics Studies

A lot of online medical companies have sprung up both at home and overseas. To select Internet medical companies or medical companies which provide online healthcare services in China and America, the author searches on the Internet with the keywords "American online healthcare company", "Internet medical" and "中国互联网医疗公司" (Chinese online healthcare company), etc. Six and five companies that appear on the top list on Google and Baidu were selected respectively. Most of the selected companies in this study are listed companies, such as PING AN Good Doctor, Longmaster and Ali Health in China, and SteadyMD, Teladoc, IQVIA, Doctor On Demand and Evolent in America. All the companies have had a wide impact on the online healthcare industry for years. The author notices that the news and blogs released on the official or relevant websites of these companies furnish abundant information about the latest services they launched, to introduce and promote their online healthcare services. The author selects 60 pieces of texts whose contents related to "online or Internet healthcare services" on "press", "newsroom" and "news and events" pages of American medical companies' websites and on "新闻动态", "公司动态" and "媒体关注" pages of Chinese medical companies' websites, including 30 pieces in Chinese and 30 pieces in English, to form a Chinese and English corpus for this study, and relevant data can be seen in Table 5-1.

Table 5-1   List of Chinese and English data

Texts	Company name	Amount of texts	Text Numbers	Total
CTs	平安好医生 PING AN Good Doctor	10	CT1-CT10	30
	阿里健康 Alibaba Health	7	CT11-CT17	
	京东健康 JD Health	6	CT18-CT23	
	春雨医生 Chunyu Doctor	1	CT24	
	微医 WeDoctor	4	CT25-CT28	
	朗玛信息 Longmaster	2	CT29-CT30	
ETs	SteadyMD	4	ET1-ET4	30
	Teladoc	13	ET5-ET17	
	Evolent	3	ET18-ET20	
	Doctor On Demand	2	ET21-ET22	
	IQVIA	8	ET23-ET30	

Some of the selected companies have been established for decades and many related online healthcare services have been launched. However, in order to maintain the timeliness of the study, the author browsed all the news pages of these companies dated from 1 May, 2018 to 31 December, 2020, selecting the corresponding texts as data by searching keywords and browsing headlines. The keywords of "launch", "complete", "expand", "establish", "develop", "collaborate", etc. in English and "达成", "启动", "落地", "搭建", "推出", "提供" etc. in Chinese are the main concerns of the author, because these words may mark the launch of a new service. Then the author conducts a second round of selection. If the headline contains relevant online healthcare service projects, it will be included into the corpus as the research target.

5.3　Cognitive Frame in Discourse Studies

As the author mentioned above, human language and cognition are inextricably linked. Namely, decoding discourse is equivalent to the process of cognitive construction, which is also called cognitive processing. Regarding the cognitive construction of discourses, cognitive linguists frequently use the concept of "cognitive frame" to analyse the linguistic devices contained in discourses and their related grammar.

5.3.1　Cognitive frame

Prior to the usage in linguistics fields, the concept of frame has been applied to computer psychology. Artificial intelligence expert Minsky (1975) argues that frame is a psychological representation of the knowledge in human world, which can be selected and extracted according to the needs of human beings. Minsky further studies how human thinking works by means of constructing mind-frames composed of pictures and languages. Fillmore (1982) introduces "frame" into linguistics, and claims that frame is a language system that reflects the cognition of the brain. He defines frame as "any system of linguistic choices—the easiest cases being collections of words, but also including choices of grammatical rules or linguistic categories—that can get associated with prototypical instances of scenes" from the perspective of language structure. For Ungerer and Schmid (2006), frame is applied to represent the knowledge and belief that is specific and appears with high frequency, which can be looked upon as a way to describe the cognitive context, playing the role of background information provider and making a connection with them. Fauconnier and Turner (1998) point out that discourse is a collection of concepts, whose meaning is the "integration" of various concepts according to certain cognitive rules which people can call it cognitive structure or cognitive frame. Discourse is the configuration of meaning, and cognitive frame is to construct and interpret the textual meaning of discourse simultaneously. As an interpretative schema, frame selectively accentuates and encodes events, objects, contexts and actions to elucidate and compress the world (Snow & Benford 1992), expecting to codify experience and guide behaviour (Snow et al. 1986). It serves as a psychological device that offers a perspective and manipulates salience to influence subsequent judgment. In discourse studies, language expressions not only highlight individual concepts, but also specify a certain perspective from which the frame is viewed. Many researchers have further explored the concepts of frame in respective fields. Among them, Rucker et al. (2008) adopt the theory of cognitive frame to study the difference in framing one-sided messages and two-sided messages. They examine how, with almost no difference in the content of a message, framing the message in different ways results in different attitudes towards the message and how to take advantage of this in message framing. Johnston and Noakes (2005) liken the process of cognitive frame construction to a "black box" (see Figure 5-1), which contains people's experiences and information they received.

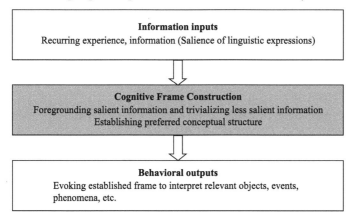

Figure 5-1   The process of cognitive frame construction (Yang et al. 2016: 9)

The information is processed in the boxes in Figure 5-1, a form which people can extract to realize and understand the world. When people get access to the world with a specific view, the optimized conceptual structure is activated and stimulated, and selection of information will promote the formation of a fixed optimization concept. To further elaborate the interrelationship between cognitive frame and linguistic devices, Yang et al. (2016) conduct a research to prove that the construction of frame could be realized by stimuli of linguistic expressions. The process of cognitive frame construction is shown in Figure 5-2.

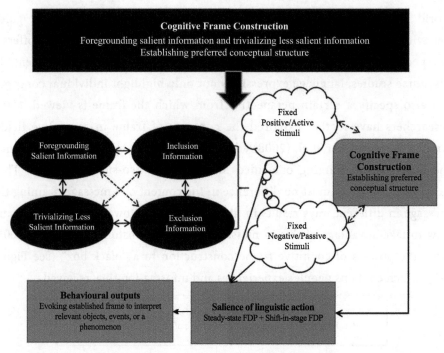

Figure 5-2　Cognitive construction and its framing process (Yang et al. 2016: 18)

From the cognitive construction and its framing process sketched in Figure 5-2, Yang et al. (2016) reveal that the stimuli of their study refer to the lexical choices which contribute to the initiation of the fixed frames and restored cognition, which can be positive, negative and even. By consciously or unconsciously choosing different information input cognitive frame, discourse constructors gradually realize their communicative purpose, and can construct the corresponding frame to interpret the surrounding events and phenomena.

In light of the above definition, interpretation and research results, cognitive frame is indeed an effective way for the study of the sense of meaning and information construction, which is also a useful tool for people to investigate the cognitive process of discourse construction.

5.3.2　Identification of move structure

5.3.2.1　Move structure

The notion of move is known to be essential to describe the features of genre, which is regarded by Swales (1990: 58) as a series of communication events shared by a discourse community with a specific communicative purpose. Sinclair and Coulthard (1975) use "move" to describe the continuous exchanges in the interactions in classrooms. Nwogu (1991) provides another definition of move: a text segment composed of a bundle of linguistic features, such as lexical meanings, prepositional meanings and illocutionary forces. Mirador (2000) defines move as "the logical manoeuvre adopted by the communicators in written or spoken discourse", fulfilling a particular purpose within the text. Swales (1990) develops a mode of *Create a Research Space* communication move structure, which consists of three moves and several steps. Cheung (2008) devises a move scheme comprising 10 major moves and 36 steps to discuss the persuasive messages in sales e-mails. Relevant to the current study on promotional genre, Bhatia (1993: 97) gives a structural interpretation assigned to sales promotional letters. He divides a sales promotional letter into seven moves, as shown in Table 5-2.

Table 5-2   **Structural interpretation of sales promotional letters (Bhatia 1993: 97)**

Move	Description	Flexibility
Move 1	establishing credentials	obligatory
Move 2	introducing the offer (i) offering the product or service (ii) essential detailing of the offer (iii) indicating value of the offer	obligatory
Move 3	offering incentives	optional
Move 4	enclosing documents	optional
Move 5	soliciting response	obligatory
Move 6	using pressure tactics	optional
Move 7	ending politely	optional

It is necessary to note that Bhatia (1993) states that the move structure of sales promotional letters is flexible, which means not all moves appear in a fixed order, nor do all sales promotional letters have to contain all seven moves he proposed. He states that Move 1 is obligatory for a sales promotional letter, which normally appears at the beginning of a text. In some cases, Move 2 will be placed at the front of Move 1 to open the letter in which the content of the letter is promoting a new product. To be general, Move 2, which is comprised of (i) offering the product or service, (ii) essential detailing of the offer and (iii) indicating value of the offer, is the most fundamental part of a letter. It should be noted that (iii) sometimes does not form a separate unit by itself but disperses around (ii). As for Move 3, Bhatia considers that it should be seen as regional rather than universal, because the resources of research data he has used include Singapore in which Move 3 is widely used but not internationally. Move 4 is also an optional unit and will be used by some enterprises to cater to their sales philosophy. Move 5 is obligatory and is just as important as Move 2. Move 6 is also optional which is decided by the products and business cultures of the enterprise. Now and then, a sales promotional letter could end with Move 5 or Move 6, but Bhatia proves that Move 7 is always the formal end of a letter.

With the evolution of promotional genre analysis, Bhatia's move structure model is not adequate to deal with more types of promotional discourses. Based on Bhatia's structure, Wang and Guo (2006: 33-34) propose a ten-move model of promotional discourses with a corpus consisting of 30 blurbs, 30 printed advertisements, 20 sales letters and 20 job applications. They try to explore the generic similarities and differences among the four types of promotional texts, as shown in Table 5-3.

Table 5-3　General move patterns of promotional texts (Wang & Guo 2006)

Move	Description
Move 1	headlines
Move 2	establishing credentials Step 2A: establishing a territory Step 2B: establishing a niche Step 2C: reestablishing business contact Step 2D: expressing gratitude Step 2E: referring to the source of job information
Move 3	introducing the offer Step 3A: offering Step 3B: essential detailing Step 3C: indicating value

continued

Move	Description
Move 4	endorsements/testimonials
Move 5	brief biography of the author or editor
Move 6	enclosing documents
Move 7	offering incentives
Move 8	using pressure tactics
Move 9	soliciting response
Move 10	ending politely

Compared with Bhatia, the numbers of move have increased to ten in Wang and Guo's research, and two of the moves are subdivided into several steps, the subordinate units of a move. The ten-move model is applicable to more types of promotional genres. In this chapter, the author refers to the move model proposed by Bhatia (1993) to identify specific move structures of Chinese and American promotional discourses of online healthcare services, and to examine how the communicative purposes have been achieved.

5.3.2.2   Moves identified in the online treatment promotional discourses

Drawing inspiration from the move structure model of promotional genre proposed by Bhatia (see Table 5-2), the author analyses 30 Chinese and English texts respectively in the corpus. However, because the corpus Bhatia studies is on sales letters, which have similarities concerning the data in this chapter on service promotions but are still different in essence, not all seven moves he proposes can be applied in this study. Move 4, for instance, "enclosing documents" does not appear in the data of the discourses here. The move structure model used in this chapter is derived from Bhatia but is not restricted by his work. The author will identify the real moves according to the actual situation of the data gathered, and delete or add some moves from Bhatia's original seven-move. After completing the analysis of 30 texts, the author obtains a seven-move structure of Chinese promotional discourses of online healthcare services, as shown in Table 5-4.

Table 5-4   Generic move structure of Chinese texts

Move	Description	Flexibility
Move 1	headline	obligatory
Move 2	establishing backgrounds	optional
Move 3	introducing the offer Step (a): offering the service or product Step (b): essential detailing Step (c): indicating value	obligatory
Move 4	establishing credentials	optional
Move 5	endorsement/testimonials	optional
Move 6	delivering performance	optional
Move 7	looking into the future	optional

Similarly studying the English promotional discourses, an eight-move structure of English promotional discourses of online healthcare services has been obtained, as shown in Table 5-5.

Table 5-5   Generic move structure of English texts

Move	Description	Flexibility
Move 1	headline	obligatory
Move 2	introductory remarks	optional
Move 3	establishing credentials	optional
Move 4	introducing the offer Step (a): offering the service or product Step (b): essential detailing Step (c): indicating value	obligatory
Move 5	establishing backgrounds	optional
Move 6	endorsement/testimonials	optional
Move 7	offering incentives	optional
Move 8	soliciting response	optional

All the moves in Chinese and English promotional discourses are identified separately. All the works are to pave the way to make further comparisons of the two kinds of discourses and then come up with some cross-cultural inspirations. The contrastive analysis is mainly about two aspects, different moves and communicative purposes. These two aspects can be discussed together because communicative purposes are fulfilled through texts with a traditional internal structure. Texts can be described as a sequence of "moves", each of which has a specific communicative purpose. Table 5-6 illustrates all the possible moves that exist in Chinese and English promotional discourses.

Table 5-6 Move comparison between Chinese and English promotional discourses

Texts	M1	M2	M3	M4	M5	M6	M7	M8
CTs	HL	EB	IO	EC	ET	DP	LF	—
ETs	HL	IR	EC	IO	EB	ET	OI	SR

Notes: In the figures throughout this book, M means move, HL means headline, EB means establishing backgrounds, IO means introducing the offer, EC means establishing credentials, ET means endorsement/testimonials, DP means delivering performance, LF means looking into the future, IR means introductory remarks, OI means offering incentives, and SR means soliciting responses.

From Table 5-6, it can be concluded that some moves such as HL, IO, EB and EC are common to the Chinese and English promotional discourses, with differences in the frequency and sequence in which they appear. The move IR exists in English texts but not in Chinese texts, which is due to Westerners' writing habit in writing press releases or corporate blogs. Another difference lies in the contact way or web page of the company that is usually attached at the end of the English texts, which is regarded as the last move SR. This can induce readers and intended consumers to learn more about the service or the whole company.

In the above analyses in this chapter, the author argues that the communicative purposes are fulfilled through different moves. Since Chinese and English promotional discourses have different move structures, the communicative purposes they desire to achieve are not the same. By comparison, it can be drawn that Chinese discourse producers take up more space to establish credentials of the company than American ones when constructing discourses. Chinese writers are more obsessed with building a good corporate image by presenting what the company has achieved. American writers, on the other hand, focus more on the introduction of their products when constructing discourses. In the move "introducing the offer", Step (b) "essential detailing" of the English texts accounts for the largest proportion, while in Chinese texts, Step (c) "indicating value" appears equally frequently.

Upton and Cohen (2009: 588) point out that "the overall discourse structure of a text can be described in relation to the sequence of move types". This is also the purpose of the author to conduct move structure analysis to identify how the writers construct a discourse from the macro level by studying the structure of a discourse. In the next section, the author will further analyse force dynamics, a typical cognitive grammar phenomenon, in Chinese and English promotional discourses.

5.4　Force Dynamics in Cognitive Frame

Interacting with the society or in the society requires the exertion of force (Yang et al. 2016: 7). Johnson (1987) claims that such force is everywhere, and our daily reality is one massive series of forceful causal sequences. Consequently, in order to comprehend our experience, we have to recognize the importance of structures of force. In addition to their role in perception and action, forces and force dynamics have many abstract metaphorical uses, e.g. conceptualizations of human emotion (Kövecses 2006), morality (Johnson 1993; Lakoff 2002), argumentation (Turner 1991), and much psychology after Freud as well as folk-psychology and metaphorical self-concepts to do with object control (Lakoff & Johnson 1999). Abstract ideas can thus be grounded in what it means to propel, arrest, divert, or enable to move physical objects or one's body. In the following, the author will explain in detail the basic patterns of force dynamics.

5.4.1　Steady-state force-dynamic patterns

As described above, Talmy's (2000) force-dynamic pattern is a description of the interaction between two force entities. Figure 5-3 presents the basic force-dynamic patterns existing in language expressions, which are known as steady-state force-dynamic patterns.

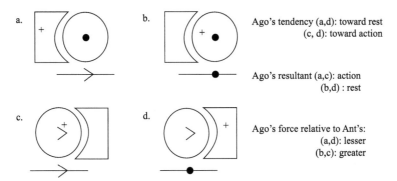

Figure 5-3 **The basic steady-state force-dynamic patterns (Talmy 2000: 415)**

Steady-state force-dynamic patterns are used to describe the possible states in which Ago may occur when Ant continuously exerts force over it, resulting in the change of the state of Ago, which includes four types: from rest to forced action, from action to forced rest, continue to move or stay rest. We should pay attention to the initial force tendency of Ago and then identify the degree of each force. The four patterns (a), (b), (c) and (d) in Figure 5-3 can be explained in the following sentences.

> a. The ball kept rolling because of the wind blowing on it.
> b. The shed kept standing despite the gale wind blowing against it.
> c. The ball kept rolling despite the stiff grass.
> d. The log kept lying on the incline because of the ridge there.

In (a), the initial intrinsic force tendency of Ago, i.e. the ball, is toward rest, but the force of Ant, i.e. the wind, is stronger than Ago and the stronger force keeps the ball in motion. This structure could be reflected in the causative structure in English. Similarly, the structure of (d) is the initial intrinsic force of Ago, the log, is toward action, but the force of Ant, the ridge, is stronger than Ago so the motion state of Ago is stopped and becomes rest. (d) is also belonging to causative structure and both (a) and (d) employ "because of", one of the marked words of causative structure. As to (b) and (c), the two structures are parts of the "despite" category in English. In (b), the initial tendency of Ago, the shed, is toward rest and its force is stronger than the opposite force exerted by Ant, so Ago is able to show its intrinsic tendency of force and remain in place. Likewise, the initial intrinsic force of Ago in (c), the ball, is toward action, although it has been obstructed by Ant, the force tendency of Ago is still realized because it has a stronger force. The force of the Ago and basic steady-state force-dynamic patterns are interpreted in Table 5-7.

Table 5-7   Basic steady-state force-dynamic patterns

Force of the Ago	Greater (Despite)	a. The ball kept rolling because of the wind blowing on it.	b. The shed kept standing despite the gale wind blowing against it.
	Lesser (Causation)	c. The ball kept rolling despite the stiff grass.	d. The log kept lying on the incline because of the ridge there.
Description		Action	Rest
Steady-state force-dynamic patterns		Tendency	

5.4.2 Shift-in-state force-dynamic patterns

Sometimes Ant does not exert force continuously over Ago, but is suddenly impacted by an external force or the force suddenly disappears. In Figure 5-4, the arrow indicates the sudden application or disappearance of a force, and the diagonal line indicates a change in motion state.

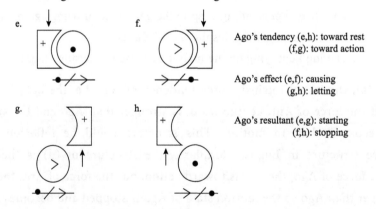

Figure 5-4   Shift-in-state force-dynamic patterns (Talmy 2000: 418)

The four patterns (e), (f), (g) and (h) in Figure 5-4 can be expressed in the following sentences.

e. The ball's hitting it made the lamp topple from the table.

f. The water's dripping on it made the fire die down.

g. The plug's coming loose let the water drain from the tank.

h. The stirring rod's breaking let the ingredients settle to the bottom.

In (e), Ant is suddenly impacted by an external force, which causes Ago to change from the rest state to the motion state. While in (f), the state of Ago is just the opposite and changes from the motion state to rest. In (g), the sudden disappearance of Ant causes Ago to change from a static state to a moving state. While in (h), the state of Ago is the opposite to (g) and the motion state is toward rest. Based on Talmy's (1988) suggestion, the shift-in-state force-dynamic patterns are interpreted in Table 5-8.

Table 5-8 Shift-in-state force-dynamic patterns

Force	starting, causing	e. A gust of wind made the pages of my book turn.	f. The appearance of the headmaster made the pupils calm down.
	stopping, letting	g. The breaking of the dam let the water flow from the storage lake.	h. The abating of the wind let the sailboat slow down.
Description		Action	Rest
Shift-in-state force-dynamic patterns		Tendency	

5.4.3 Secondary steady-state force-dynamic patterns

The last pattern is secondary steady-state force-dynamic patterns (see Figure 5-5). In this pattern, the force exerted on the Ago does not occur suddenly, but remains away constantly. Therefore, the initial state of Ago is possibly staying the same. To some extent, secondary steady-state force-dynamic patterns are similar to steady-state force-dynamic patterns.

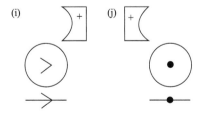

Figure 5-5 Secondary steady-state force-dynamic patterns (Talmy 2000: 420)

The influence of Ant exerts on Ago is not sudden, but remains constant. The slight difference between the two patterns is that in secondary steady-state force-dynamic patterns, however strong or weak the force of Ant, it has little influence on Ago. Therefore, steady-state force-dynamic patterns are often omitted in the study of force-dynamic model.

Kimmel (2011) further extends the theory from the previous version to the field of literature from Text-Linguistics to Literary-Actants in the Force Dynamics of Vampirism. This theory is applied to classify the emotional processes in the novel through computer assisting quantitative cumulative system (CAQCS) to calculate the numbers of his specific classification over several basic force-dynamic patterns based on his sorting out patterns. It is necessary to determine what is to concern. A useful first question is "Who are the conceptualized agents? ", i.e. who is singled out for focal attention and in relation to whom. Once we have determined agonist and antagonist, it makes sense to chart the basic force tendencies of a protagonist (temporary or lasting) across specific interactions. The next question is "What roles do the agents take on face to face each other? " In another empirical research on media discourses of China rail promotional reports, Yang et al (2016) point out that some marked words such as "despite" category in (b) and (c) in force-dynamic pattern could be seen as an active linguistic stimulus which can realize the force of Ago. In contrast, "because of" as the "causative" kind in (a) and (d) should be regarded as the passive linguistic stimuli for the force realization of Ago. Language expressions, especially stimulus, can reflect and structure human cognition and its framing processes. As mentioned before, stimuli refer to the lexical choices which contribute to the initiation of the fixed frames and restored cognition (Yang et al. 2020). Force dynamics is an effective approach to identifying the stimuli that exist in discourses. The author intends to demystify how linguistic stimuli reflect discourse producers' cognition when engaged in promotional discourse writing. This analysis helps to reveal the complicated relationship between language expression and cognition.

5.5　Force Dynamics in Promotional Discourses of Online Treatments

After completing the discourse analysis from the macro/discoursal level, the second half of the data analysis will be carried out from the micro/semantic level. Drawing insights from force-dynamic theory proposed by Talmy (2000), the author intends to delve into what linguistic selections of force-dynamics are employed in Chinese and English promotional discourses, and to illustrate the cognitive frames and their framing processes. When Yang et al. (2016) study the cognitive frame construction of foreign media on Chinese high-speed railway news reports, they divide the research targets into the pattern with stronger Antagonist (Antagonist+/Ant+) and the pattern with stronger Agonist (Agonist+/Ago+) on the basis of the three force-dynamic patterns proposed by Talmy (2000). The criterion for this classification is the strength of Ant and Ago. The author will follow this classification criterion when carrying out the analysis of this chapter, selecting the linguistic devices related to the representations of force-dynamic patterns and their schemas. By investigating how these patterns are externalized in linguistic data, we could get to know how the cognitive frames of discourse producers promoting their online healthcare services are constructed in the Chinese and English promotional discourses.

5.5.1 Analysis of force-dynamic elements in Chinese discourses

With regard to force-dynamic theory, its three major patterns and elements have been represented in previous Chapter 3. In line with the two classifications of "**Antagonist+**" and "**Agonist+**" ('+' refers to a stronger force), the author will dissect the force-dynamic elements of linguistic selections in Chinese promotional discourses.

5.5.1.1 "Antagonist+" pattern

"Antagonist+" pattern consists mainly of (a) and (d) of the basic steady-state force-dynamic patterns (see Figure 5-3), and four shift-in-state force-dynamic patterns (see Figure 5-4). In "Antagonist+" pattern, the initial force of Ago is weaker than that of Ant. Imposing on Ant, Ago cannot maintain its intrinsic tendency and begin to change; or gradually returns to its initial motion state when the force of a stronger Ant is loosed or removed suddenly. Yang et al. (2016) argue that in this "Antagonist+" pattern, a positive stimulus is generated in these two force-interacting entities. The positive stimuli referring to the change in the motion state of Ago are caused by the force exerted by Ant.

Example 14 (Source: CT6)

规范化诊疗以及长期个体化的健康管理方案[Ant]，可以做到精准筛查，也可以大大阻止病情[Ago]进一步恶化，提高慢阻肺患者生活质量。（平安好医生与勃林格殷格翰深度合作，打造中国首个线上慢阻肺全方位管理项目，平安好医生/勃林格殷格翰，2020 年 7 月 9 日）①

Standardized treatment and long-term individualized health management programs [Ant] can achieve accurate screening and greatly **prevent** further deterioration of the sickness [Ago], improving the life quality of COPD (Chronic Obstructive Pulmonary Disease) patients. (PING AN Good Doctor and Boehringer Ingelheim have cooperated deeply to create China's first online COPD comprehensive management project, PING AN Good Doctor/ Boehringer Ingelheim, 9 July, 2020)

Example 15 (Source: CT7)

平安好医生推出的创新型互联网医疗模式[Ant] "名医工作室"，针对这些问题[Ago]提供专业的方案。（名医工作室上线！15 位名医成为首批平安好医生名医合伙人，平安好医生/新浪财经，2020 年 8 月 17 日）②

"Famous Doctor Studio", an innovative Internet medical model [Ant] launched by PING AN Good Doctor, **provides** professional **solutions** to these problem [Ago]. (Famous doctor studio online! Fifteen famous doctors became the first batch of PING AN Good Doctor Famous Doctor partners, PING AN Good Doctor/SINA Finance, 17 August, 2020)

The force-dynamic pattern contained in these two examples is **(d) pattern** (see Figure 5-6) of the basic steady-state force-dynamic patterns in which the force of Ant is stronger in two interactive entities, and Ago does not realize its intrinsic tendency towards action. There is a positive stimulus between Ant and Ago, which causes the motion state of Ago to become rest. In Example 14, the stronger force is the health management program offered by the medical company which can effectively prevent the sickness. It is meant to stop the

① https://www.boehringer-ingelheim.cn/press-releases/ping-an-hao-yi-sheng-yu-bo-lin-ge-yin-ge-han-shen-du-he-zuo-da-zao-zhong-guo-shou-ge-xian-shang-man-zu-fei-quan-fang-wei-guan-li-xiang-mu

② https://finance.sina.com.cn/wm/2020-08-17/doc-iivhvpwy1525976.shtml

progression of COPD, a chronic sickness. Until then, the intrinsic tendency of Ago is towards action, but it cannot continue to keep the initial motion state and gradually towards rest because of the opposing force, as well as a positive stimulus, exerted by Ant. In a similar way, the innovative Internet medical model launched by the company is also the stronger force in Example 15. The introduction of it has succeeded in preventing some of the problems in the current medical situation, including the lack of individual brand building ability and an unbalanced distribution of medical resources. Ant has again changed the intrinsic tendency of Ago due to its stronger force, making Ago impossible to realize its initial motion state towards action.

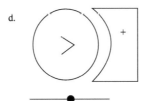

Figure 5-6   Steady-state force-dynamic pattern (d)

Example 16 (Source: CT5)

随着大健康产业的飞速发展和养生观念的年轻化，消费者对草本食品类产品需求[Ago]愈发强烈。（平安好医生牵手津村（中国）互联网医疗赋能中药材供应链，中国新闻网，2020 年 12 月 16 日）①

With the rapid development of Comprehensive Health Industry and the rejuvenation of health preservation, the demand for herbal food products [Ago] of consumers is increasingly growing. (PING AN Good Doctor and Tsumura (China) have reached a strategic cooperation on the Internet medical enabling Chinese herbal medicine supply chain, ChinaNews.com, 16 December, 2020)

Example 17 (Source: CT5)

此次合作的达成，平安好医生为津村打开了将日本当地特色产品引入中国[Ago]的窗口，为国内消费者提供更丰富的药品。（平安好医生牵手津村（中国）互联网医疗赋能中药材供应链，中国新闻网，2020 年 12 月 16 日）②

---

① https://www.chinanews.com.cn/business/2020/12-16/9363484.shtml
② https://www.chinanews.com.cn/business/2020/12-16/9363484.shtml

With this cooperation, PING AN Good Doctor **opened a window for** Tsumura <u>to introduce local products from Japan to China</u> [Ago], providing more abundant drugs for domestic consumers. (PING AN Good Doctor and Tsumura (China) have reached a strategic cooperation on the Internet medical enabling Chinese herbal medicine supply chain, ChinaNews.com, 16 December, 2020)

The force-dynamic pattern contained in these two examples is **(e) pattern** (see Figure 5-7) of shift-in-state force-dynamic patterns. A stronger force enters to cause the state of Ago shifting from rest to action. The force of Ago is still weak and changed by the entry of a strong force. In Example 16, the rapid development of comprehensive health industry and rejuvenation of health preservation are the stronger force entered. Even consumers tend to demand herbal foods before, the motion state of it is initially rest. The state of Ago changed from rest to action after the entry of a stronger force. The demand for herbal products begins to grow stronger. Example 17 is the same, due to the external force, the cooperation of two companies, Japanese local products could be manufactured in China. The process which has a state of transition from rest to action contains a "causative" relationship between Ago and Ant.

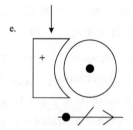

Figure 5-7　Shift-in-state force-dynamic pattern (e)

Example 18 (Source: CT22)

依托京东健康平台优质的产品资源, <u>缓解医院看病的压力</u> [Ago]。(京东健康联合中国联通推出"抗击冠状病毒 线上健康支援"活动, 京东健康, 2020 年 2 月 5 日) ①

Relying on the high-quality product resources of JD Health to **relieve** <u>the pressure of hospital treatment</u> [Ago]. (JD Health and China Unicom

---

① http://www.techweb.com.cn/internet/2020-02-05/2775721.shtml

launched the campaign of "online health support against coronavirus", JD Health, 5 February, 2020)

Example 19 (Source: CT7)

伴随着国家层面的决策利好，用户在线问诊习惯的快速养成，<u>诸多医疗痛点[Ago]有望被逐一攻克</u>。（名医工作室上线！15 位名医成为首批平安好医生名医合伙人，平安好医生/新浪财经，2020 年 8 月 17 日）①

With the favourable decision-making at the national level and the rapid formation of users' online consultation habits, <u>several medical pain points</u> [Ago] are expected to be **overcome** one by one. (Famous doctor studio online! Fifteen famous doctors became the first batch of PING AN Good Doctor Famous Doctor partners, PING AN Good Doctor/SINA Finance, 17 August, 2020)

The force-dynamic pattern contained in these two examples is **(f) pattern** (see Figure 5-8) of shift-in-state force-dynamic patterns. In this pattern, a stronger force enters to cause the motion state of Ago to change from action to rest. The weaker Ago comes to a halt because of the entering of a stronger Ant force. In Examples 18 and 19, the function of stronger force is embodied in terms of "缓解" (relieve) and "攻克" (overcome) that vividly embody a process from action to rest. Stress and pain points gradually realize their tendency towards rest with the force of high-quality resources and favourable policies.

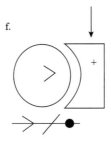

Figure 5-8   Shift-in-state force-dynamic pattern (f)

From the above analysis, it can be seen that in **"Antagonist+" pattern**, Ant is foregrounded, and the information about Ant is constantly highlighted. In promotional discourses, Ant is always a good and favourable aspect, thus

---

① https://finance.sina.com.cn/wm/2020-08-17/doc-iivhvpwy1525976.shtml

the writer should continuously amplify and highlight its function and influence. As positive stimuli, they can play an active role.

5.5.1.2 "Agonist+" pattern

The main force-dynamic patterns corresponding to "Agonist+" pattern are (b) and (c) in the steady-state force-dynamic patterns (see Figures 5-9 and 5-10). In these patterns, the force of Ago is stronger than Ant, so Ago is able to maintain its initial motion state even when it is subjected to the force exerted by Ant. The force functions as a negative stimulus since it does not succeed in shifting the state of Ago. The general sentence pattern of "Agonist+" is "although Ant... Ago still...".

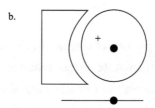

Figure 5-9　Steady-state force-dynamic pattern (b)

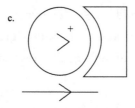

Figure 5-10　Steady-state force-dynamic pattern (c)

Example 20 (Source: CT15)

相关的临床试验在社交媒体上的宣传[Ant]有所增加，但信息毕竟有限，亦缺乏透明性，患者"招募难"问题[Ago]仍有待解决。（全球找药联盟上线，助解"药神"难题，搜狐网，2018 年 7 月 11 日）①

Related clinical trials have increased their publicity [Ant] on social media, but with limited information and a lack of transparency, the "difficulty in recruiting of patients" [Ago] **remains** to be addressed. (A platform for global drug finders launched to help solve the problem of "drug

---

① https://www.sohu.com/a/240452336_377305

god", SOHU.com, 11 July, 2018)

This example illustrates the **(b) pattern** (see Figure 5-9) of steady-state force-dynamic patterns. In this pattern, Ago is stronger and could retain its intrinsic tendency towards rest even when it is under the influence of Ant. This pattern works as a negative stimulus because the motion state of the entity does not shift. In this example, the publicity of clinical trials is an attempt to solve the recruitment problem, just as the process of Ant exerting force on Ago. However, the recruitment problem has not been resolved since Ant is not strong enough to have an impact on Ago, so Ago can retain its intrinsic tendency towards rest.

Example 21 (Source: CT7)

名医工作室[Ago]**打破**时间、空间隔阂[Ant]，给患者提供与全国顶级名医一对一线上即时交流平台。（名医工作室上线！15 位名医成为首批平安好医生名医合伙人，平安好医生/新浪财经，2020 年 8 月 17 日）①

<u>Famous doctor studio</u> [Ago] **breaks** the <u>gap of time and space</u> [Ant], providing patients with a one-to-one online instant communication platform with the top famous doctors. (Famous doctor studio online! Fifteen famous doctors became the first batch of PING AN Good Doctor Famous Doctor partners, PING AN Good Doctor/SINA Finance, 17 August, 2020)

Example 21 illustrates the **(c) pattern** of steady-state force-dynamic patterns. In pattern (c), Ago is the stronger force which is able to realize its intrinsic tendency towards action (see Figure 5-10). This pattern functions as a negative stimulus because Ago continues to move under the action of Ant. In this example, although there are no obvious signal words such as "despite" or "even though", the meaning the discourse producer intends to express can be decoded from the context. The idea of this sentence is that even with the gap in space and time, the "famous doctor studio" launched by the company still could provide patients with a platform of top doctors for one-to-one online consultations. The gap imposed on the service is not enough to prevent its initial motion state. Ant is "failure to prevent" Ago from shifting state, and this pattern

---

① https://finance.sina.com.cn/wm/2020-08-17/doc-iivhvpwy1525976.shtml

works as a negative stimulus. The intrinsic tendency of Ago is towards action and it could continue to move after bearing the force exerted by Ant.

5.5.2 Analysis of force-dynamic elements in English discourses

In the same way, the author analyses English data in accordance with the classification methods of "Antagonist+" pattern and "Agonist+" pattern. Some of the basic information has already been manifested in the analysis of force-dynamic elements in Chinese discourses, so the author directly studies the examples and omits the explanations of the force-dynamic patterns applied in the Chinese data in section 5.5.1.

5.5.2.1 "Antagonist+" pattern

Similarly, the author continues to analyse the steady-state force-dynamic patterns and shift-in-state force-dynamic patterns in English texts. The similar cases and their interpretations to Chinese ones are not repeatedly elaborated in this section but distinct linguistic expressions in English are selected for the following analysis.

Example 22 (Source: ET6)
This limited patient support, coupled with a strained healthcare system and long wait times [Ant], has **resulted in** an absence of care [Ago] for rural Aboriginal communities in Canada. (350+ Indigenous organizations to benefit from Teladoc Health telemedicine services, Teladoc, 10 June, 2020) [①]

The force-dynamic pattern manifested in Example 22 is **(a) pattern** of the basic steady-state force-dynamic patterns in which the force of Ant is stronger in two interactive entities, and Ago does not realize its intrinsic tendency towards rest and begins to move (see Figure 5-11). Ago fails to resist the force exerted by Ant. In this example, "an absence of care" was originally a stationary state, or it didn't exist in the first place. But the limited patient support and other factors contributed to the region begins to lack of medical care, and the entity that is initially inclined to rest is forced to move. There is a "causative"

---

① https://s21.q4cdn.com/672268105/files/doc_news/350-Indigenous-organizations-to-benefit-from-Teladoc-Health-telemedicine-services-2020.pdf

relationship between Ant and Ago and works as a positive stimulus to shift the motion state of Ago.

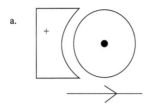

Figure 5-11 Steady-state force-dynamic pattern (a)

Example 23 (Source: ET3)

COVID-19 is at the fore-front but major <u>healthcare problems</u> [Ago] related to chronic disease, lack of access to care and other health care challenges, can be more effectively **addressed with** <u>continuous care</u> [Ant]. (SteadyMD Telemedicine Doctors Provide Alternative to Face-to-Face Clinical Visits for COVID-19 Concerns, SteadyMD, 11 March, 2020)[1]

Example 24 (Source: ET25)

<u>A new cloud-based software as a service (SaaS) solution</u> [Ant] that helps **close** <u>the gap</u> [Ago] between life sciences companies and patients. (IQVIA Launches Orchestrated Patient Engagement, IQVIA, 2 October, 2019)[2]

Example 25 (Source: ET6)

<u>Teladoc Health telemedicine services</u> [Ant] will help more than 350 First Nations and Inuit employers **close** <u>gaps in care access for their employees</u> [Ago]. (350+ Indigenous organizations to benefit from Teladoc Health telemedicine services, Teladoc, 10 June, 2020)[3]

The force-dynamic pattern manifested in Examples 23, 24, 25 is **(d) pattern** of the basic steady-state force-dynamic pattern. In the three examples, Ago presents something negative, such as healthcare problems and gaps that already exist (see Figure 5-12). The initial state of Ago is action until the force applied from Ant is received. However, due to a stronger force from Ant, such

---

[1] https://www.steadymd.com/2020/03/11/steadymd-telemedicine-doctors-provide-alternative-to-face-to-face-clinical-visits-for-covid-19-concerns/

[2] https://www.iqvia.com/zh-cn/newsroom/2019/10/iqvia-launches-orchestrated-patient-engagement

[3] https://s21.q4cdn.com/672268105/files/doc_news/350-Indigenous-organizations-to-benefit-from-Teladoc-Health-telemedicine-services-2020.pdf

as "continuous care" in Example 23, "a new cloud-based software" in Example 24 and "telemedicine services" in Example 25, the state of Ago is forced to shift from previous action to rest. Because all the three Ant expressions play positive roles in problem-solving and gap-filling, there is a "causative" relation between Ant and Ago, which also functions as a positive stimulus.

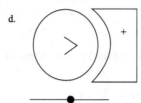

Figure 5-12　Steady-state force-dynamic pattern (d)

Example 26 (Source: ET22)

With the population aging and the prevalence of chronic disease growing, <u>enormous burdens</u> [Ago] on medicine, especially primary care, are **rising**. (Doctor On Demand Launches Synapse, a New Virtual Care Platform Delivering Next Generation Primary Care for Health Plan and Employer Populations, Doctor On Demand, 26 February, 2019)[1]

Example 27 (Source: ET2)

<u>Telehealth visits</u> [Ago] are **booming** as doctors and patients embrace distancing amid the coronavirus crisis. (SteadyMD Collaborates with CareDash to Match Doctors with People Nationwide for Online Care, SteadyMD, 19 May, 2020)[2]

The force-dynamic pattern contained in these two examples is **(e) pattern** of shift-in-state force-dynamic patterns. A stronger force enters to cause the state of Ago changing from rest to action (see Figure 5-13). In Example 26, population aging and the prevalence of chronic disease are the stronger forces entering the scenario, resulting in the burden becoming obvious and increasing gradually. Ago cannot realize its intrinsic tendency towards rest and is forced to change to action under the impact of external forces. In

---

[1]　https://www.businesswire.com/news/home/20190226005249/en

[2]　https://www.steadymd.com/blog/steadymd-collaborates-with-caredash-to-match-doctors-with-people-nationwide-for-online-care/

Example 27, the external force is derived from the objective need for doctors and patients to keep their distance during the virus crisis. Accordingly, telehealth visits as the Ago are affected, resulting in its state from the initial rest to action.

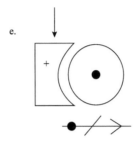

Figure 5-13   Shift-in-state force-dynamic pattern (e)

Example 28 (Source: ET11)

With this new addition to the Teladoc Health care continuum, patients and employers can now leverage virtual care to **reduce** the intensity, frustration and impact of back pain [Ago]. (Teladoc Health Expands Continuum of Services with Addition of Back Care Solution, Teladoc, 17 January, 2019)[1]

Example 29 (Source: ET16)

In line with these trends, the new integrated app experience enables members to meet their care needs along a spectrum of conditions, whenever and wherever they are, **removing** the complexity of accessing care [Ago]. (Teladoc Announces Commercial Availability of Integrated Teladoc—Best Doctors Mobile App Experience, Teladoc, 9 January, 2018)[2]

The force-dynamic pattern contained in these two examples is **(f) pattern** of shift-in-state force-dynamic patterns. Actually, the elements of this pattern are very similar to that of (e) pattern (see Figure 5-14). Both patterns have a stronger force exerting on Ago and change their states by the positive stimulus. The difference is that in (e) pattern the Ago is forced to move, whereas in this

---

[1] https://business.teladochealth.com/newsroom/press/release/Teladoc-Health-Expands-Continuum-of-Services-with-Addition-of-Back-Care-Solution-01-17-2019/

[2] https://business.teladochealth.com/newsroom/press/release/Teladoc-Announces-Commercial-Availability-of-Integrated-Teladoc---Best-Doctors-Mobile-App-Experience-01-09-2018/

pattern the Ago stops moving because of strong resistance. In Examples 28 and 29, the state of Ago is changed from action to rest after being affected by external forces. The two verbs "reduce" and "remove" could depict the changing process.

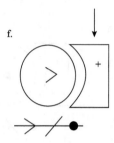

Figure 5-14   Shift-in-state force-dynamic pattern (f)

5.5.2.2   "Agonist+" pattern

In English texts, discourse writers also use "Agonist+" pattern expressions to present negative stimuli owing to their failure in changing the force of Ago entities.

Example 30 (Source: ET11)

Back pain [Ago] also is known to have **low adherence to** <u>traditional</u> <u>therapy and treatment options</u> [Ant]. (Teladoc Health Expands Continuum of Services with Addition of Back Care Solution, Teladoc, 17 January, 2019)[①]

Example 30 depicts **(b) pattern** of the basic steady-state force-dynamic patterns. Ago is stronger and can remain its intrinsic tendency towards rest even when it is under the influence of Ant (see Figure 5-15). This pattern works as a negative stimulus because the motion state of the entity does not shift. In this example, the intrinsic tendency of Ago is towards rest since the "back pain" has persisted. The other of the interactive entities is "traditional therapy", which has a weaker force than back pain. Thus, the force exerted by the weaker Ant cannot make Ago change its state. The problem with back pain

---

① https://s21.q4cdn.com/672268105/files/doc_news/Teladoc-Health-Expands-Continuum-of-Services-with-Addition-of--Back-Care-Solution.pdf

is not solved by traditional therapy, so Ago is able to realize its intrinsic tendency towards rest.

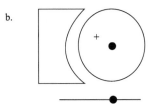

Figure 5-15   Steady-state force-dynamic pattern (b)

Example 31 (Source: ET13)

With this <u>unique service</u> [Ago], a state-licensed doctor works directly with individuals, **regardless of** <u>their geographic location</u> [Ant], to get timely answers regarding accurate diagnoses and treatment plans advice. (Teladoc Health Launches Teladoc Medical Experts for Complex Physical and Mental Health Conditions, 25 October, 2019)[①]

Example 31 depicts **(c) pattern** of the basic steady-state force-dynamic patterns. In pattern (c), Ago is the stronger force which is able to realize its intrinsic tendency towards action (see Figure 5-16). This pattern functions as a negative stimulus because Ago continues to move under the action of Ant. The "unique service" in this excerpt is actually limited by geographical locations, which is an objective existence. But the force of it is weaker than the unique service. In other words, the unique service is still able to function well despite the geographical limitations. So Ago could maintain its intrinsic tendency towards action.

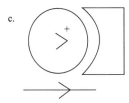

Figure 5-16   Steady-state force-dynamic pattern (c)

[①]   https://business.teladochealth.com/newsroom/press/release/Teladoc-Health-Launches-Teladoc-Medical-Experts-for-Complex-Physical-and-Mental-Health-Conditions-10-25-2019/

5.6 Cross-cultural Differences of Force Dynamics in Promotional Discourses of Online Treatments

Through the separate analysis, it can be drawn that there is a commonality that force-dynamic patterns exist in both Chinese and English promotional discourses of online healthcare services, that is, discourse producers are more inclined to use "Antagonist+" pattern to make expressions. Based on the examples given in the first two sections, the author lists Antagonist, Agonist and marked words in different patterns respectively, which present the similarities and differences concerning the linguistic selections and their embodied force dynamics in both Chinese and English promotional discourses of online healthcare services (see Table 5-9).

Table 5-9   Force-dynamic elements in Chinese and English promotional discourses

	Pattern	Antagonist	Agonist	Marked words
CTs	Ant+ (d)	health management programs; innovative Internet medical model	illness; problems	prevent; provide solutions
	Ant+ (e)	rapid development; cooperation	demand; local products	with...
	Ant+ (f)	favorable policy; high-quality product resources	pressure; pain points	relieve; overcome
	Ago+ (b)	publicity	difficulty	remain
	Ago+ (c)	gap	service project	break
ETs	Ant+ (a)	limited supports	absence of care	resulted in
	Ant+ (d)	continuous care;solution	healthcare problems; gap	address; close
	Ant+ (e)	population aging	burdens	with...
	Ant+ (f)	health care; new app	pain; complexity	reduce; remove
	Ago+ (b)	traditional therapy	pain	low adherence to
	Ago+ (c)	geographic location	service	regardless of

"Antagonist+" pattern is to foreground the Ant of two "force-interacting entities" in force-dynamic pattern, that is, to constantly amplify and highlight the roles and functions of Antagonist. As we can see from Table 5-9, most of the entities that belong to Ago are negative in "Antagonist+" pattern, such as problems, pressures and gaps. While the foregrounded Ant is always good and positive, for example, the latest service launched by the company or new cooperation with other companies. Especially in Chinese discourses, almost all Antagonists are good aspects.

It is not surprising that discourse producers more often use Antagonist+ pattern when writing promotional discourses. Because one of the main purposes of writing promotional discourse is to highlight the advantages and value of the product or service, this force dynamic pattern could meet such a need. In the first part of the move structure analysis, the author has mentioned that in the English data, discourse producers pay more attention to the detailed description of the service which might have an invisible requirement of the treatment, so flat-out language is preferred for them.

According to the analytical procedures of this study, the author first divides the promotional discourses into a series of moves with different communicative purposes, and then summarizes the generic move structure of Chinese and English promotional discourses of online healthcare services respectively. Force-dynamic analysis is conducted based on the move structure analysis. The author distinguishes what linguistic selections are employed by discourse producers in each move, and finds out that either in Chinese or English data, the locations of these linguistic selections with "force" usually appear in Move 2 "establishing backgrounds", Move 3 "introducing the offer", and Move 4 "establishing credentials". Yang et al. (2016) hold that linguistic expressions, especially stimuli, affect the cognition of discourse consumers and their framing processes of relevant subjects and phenomena. This part of analysis uses force-dynamic theory to reveal the stimuli contained in linguistic expression, which could be positive or negative. These linguistic stimuli help readers to form a frame for comprehending subjects and phenomena in the world. In the next section, the author explores the cognitive frame of online healthcare service promotion from a semantic/micro perspective by applying force-dynamic analysis.

The two analytical procedures in this study of Chinese and English promotional discourses of online healthcare services can be seen as the processes of expounding the cognitive frame that discourse producers construct to illustrate the image of online healthcare services. Drawing insights from the process of cognitive frame construction proposed by Johnston and Noakes (2005), the author comes up with a slightly different cognitive frame construction process according to the actual research situation of this chapter as shown in Figure 5-17.

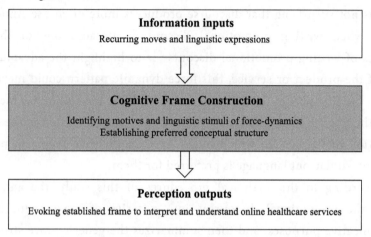

Figure 5-17　The process of cognitive frame construction in promotional discourses of this study

On the one hand, when constructing a promotional discourse, the language used by discourse producers contains certain motives, which could be identified by means of move structure analysis, because a discourse can be described as a sequence of "moves", each of which owns its special communicative purpose(s). The use of move structure to interpret the discourse structure can reveal the aspects from which the discourse producers try to introduce and promote their online healthcare services and what kind of motivation they expect to achieve, so as to construct the cognition of online healthcare services in the readers' minds. On the other hand, the author analyzes the discourse from the perspective of linguistic selection. After making clear that the discourse is composed of a sequence of "moves" and reflects various motives of discourse producers, the employment of force-dynamic expressions in promotional discourses can make readers conceptualize the target object prompted in discourses. Discourse producers arrange the information of discourses using either positive stimuli or negative stimuli to influence readers' cognition.

Different thinking patterns due to the diversity of culture and business backgrounds lead to variant ways of cognition. Although the general purpose of promotional discourses is the same, there are still discrepancies in cognition and its framing process. Based on the analysis results, the processes of cognitive frame construction of Chinese and English promotional discourses of online healthcare services are shown in Figure 5-18 and Figure 5-19.

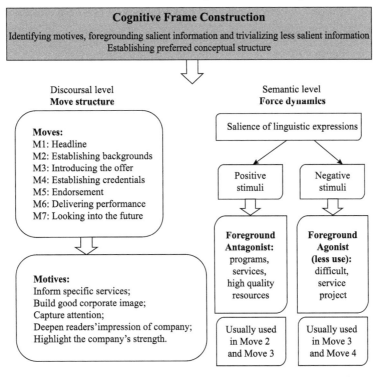

Figure 5-18　Cognitive frame construction in Chinese promotional discourses

Figure 5-18 presents the preferred cognitive frame in which the producers of Chinese online healthcare service promotional discourses expect readers to construct for the services they promote. First of all, by sorting out the discourse structure, the author obtains seven moves with different communicative purposes and finds that the motives of each move contained in Chinese discourses are more inclined to build a good corporate image in the readers' mind, and less to introduce the services they want to promote. Then the author investigates the semantic expressions, when using discourse to shape readers' cognitive image of online healthcare services. Discourse producers tend to choose positive stimuli in "Antagonist+" pattern to activate and solidify readers' positive impression of the whole service project by emphasizing the innovative mode, strength and quality projects of their companies, etc., so as to encourage readers to make choices and consumption. The description of the overall strength of the company in Chinese discourses guides readers to realize that the services are supported by reliable and guaranteed hardware conditions, which caters to the psychology of Chinese people who trust big brands more. The information about promoting services is mainly considered from the perspective of social impact and institutional expertise.

For English discourses, a different eight-move structure is obtained. Paying more attention to describing the detailed information of services from different aspects, discourse producers build a relatively abundant frame about the service itself in the readers' mind, so that the readers can have a deeper impression of the services they want to promote (see Figure 5-19). Semantically, English discourses also tend to use positive stimuli in "Antagonist+" pattern to

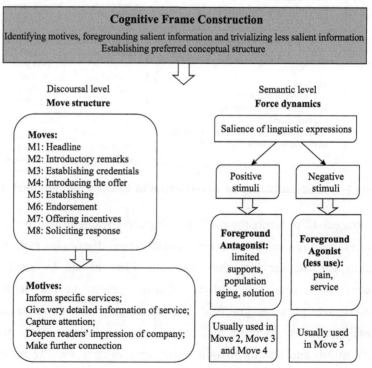

Figure 5-19   Cognitive frame construction in English promotional discourses

activate and solidify readers' positive impression of services. The information about promotion is mainly considered from the perspective of specific services and commercial intentions.

5.7   Summary

Under the framework of move structure and force dynamics, the author analyses the promotional discourses of online healthcare services in China and America from the level of discourse and semantics, and interpreted the cognitive frame contained in this kind of discourse and its constructing process. Figure 5-20 displays a generic illustration of the cognitive frame construction processes in Chinese and English promotional discourses of online healthcare services.

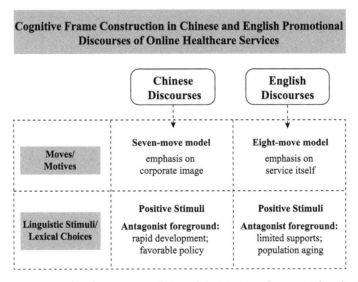

Figure 5-20   Overall Illustration of Cognitive Frame Construction in Chinese and English Promotional Discourses

Accordingly, the author gets an overall illustration of the whole process. Just as what have been discussed in sections 5.1 and 5.2, the move structures and linguistic selections of force dynamics are different in Chinese and English data. On the one hand, the author obtains a seven-move and an eight-move model from Chinese and English data respectively. Chinese texts emphasize and highlight the strength and influence of the company, while English texts prefer to focus on the service itself. On the other hand, although both Chinese and English discourse producers prefer to use positive stimuli to make expressions, the Antagonists they foreground are different. Almost all foreground Antagonists in Chinese texts are positive factors, such as favourable policies and rapid development, while English texts foreground some negative factors such as limited support. As the "black box" of human cognition construction, this process affects people's understanding and acceptance of objects and phenomena. Through data analysis and discussion, the recurring expressions in Chinese and English promotional discourses of online healthcare services reinforce readers' cognition of the promotional services, from which readers can extract information that the discourse producers want to convey and construct the corresponding cognitive frames, helping readers to understand and accept online healthcare services.

Chapter 6

Grounding Grammar in Promotional Discourses of Medical Treatment Appliances

As the growing health concern among the public requires leading medical devices, the global medical device market is gradually expanding. Meanwhile, market penetration and revenue generation propel medical device companies to be ever more competitive. The situation is much more salient in the coronary stent market which is now dominated by North American and European companies. One domestic medical device company MicroPort Scientific Corporation has gained worldwide recognition. Besides, since the average price of coronary stents is down to 700 RMB and instances of coronary diseases have gone up for some period of time, the demand for coronary stents has grown rapidly for some time. It is a good chance for other domestic medical device companies to earn their market share and build a good reputation in the international coronary market. Therefore, it entails cross-linguistic and cross-cultural communication needs.

Typically, medical device companies attract journalists, shareholders, and potential buyers' attention by releasing coronary-related news on their websites where increasing quantity and quality of information on promoting coronary stents are available to disseminate product information, maintain visibility and acquire readers. News is published online with little or no delay and is also considered as a source to promote products, values, and companies themselves. Therefore, the significance of news releases speaks for itself. There is evidence that the conscious perception and attention of East Asians and Westerners are quite different (Nisbett & Miyamoto 2005). This chapter examines the cognitive mechanisms embedded in modal use in English and Chinese medical device promotion news (hereafter MDPNs) so as to give some insights for Chinese medical device discourse producers into obtaining compliance with the target readership.

6.1 Introduction

Grounding theory is initially proposed by Langacker (1991) who further develops it into nominal and finite clause grounding in *Cognitive Grammar: A Basic Introduction* (Langacker 2008). He emphasizes how the use of grounding elements contributes to the connection between the object (entity) or event (process) and the cognitive scene in the mental space of speech event participants. In other words, the speaker relates an entity or process to the current speech event in such a way that the hearer gains cognitive access to or mental contact with the entity or process. Some core concepts are introduced as follows.

For grounding theory, clausal grounding includes tense and modal grounding. Since the news or press releases are characterized by using present tense, this study will only focus on modal grounding in discourses. In cognitive linguistics, it is generally accepted that modals are properly characterized by the concept of force dynamics. Therefore, the conceptions of physical or abstract force are reflected in the conceptualization process of modals.

6.2 Data for Modal Verb Grounding Grammar Studies

The texts analysed are mainly retrieved from the official websites of famous Chinese and American medical device companies that produce coronary stents. The medical device companies selected are listed, ranked top ten in their home market, and specialized in developing cardiovascular products. Those medical device companies ranked top ten but not specialized in developing coronary stents are excluded. The Chinese data consists of 30 texts issued by four Chinese medical device companies and the English data consists of 30 texts issued by five American medical device companies, from 1 Jan. 2014 to 31 Dec. 2020. The texts are collected systematically. First, target well-known Chinese and American medical device companies developing coronary stents on Baidu and Google respectively; second, source keywords "stent" and "coronary" to retrieve qualified press releases on companies' news pages. The topics covered in the texts are restricted to those generally positive, including updates on and results of clinical trials, commercial implementations, decisions taken by regulatory authorities, awards on certain types of products, international meetings, etc. Table 6-1 shows the data about the English and Chinese texts included.

Table 6-1   Data of the English and Chinese texts

Texts	Company names	Amount of texts	Numbers	Total
ETs	Medtronic	14	ET1-ET14	30
	Boston Scientific	5	ET15-ET19	
	Abbott Laboratories	9	ET20-ET28	
	Cardinal Health	2	ET29-ET30	
CTs	微创 (MicroPort)	17	CT1-CT17	30
	蓝帆医疗 (Bluesail Medical)	5	CT18-CT22	
	赛诺医疗 (SINOMED)	5	CT23-CT27	
	乐普医疗 (Lepu Medical)	3	CT28-CT30	

The reasons why coronary stent promotional discourses in the medical industry are chosen for this research are the favourable market environment and the particularity of this industry. The demand for coronary stents is increasing year on year because of the growing instances of coronary diseases, and healthcare insurance expands the purchasing power of citizens, and the average price of a coronary stent in China has been reduced to about 700 RMB. The market environment offers a great opportunity for Chinese companies to go global. The most cost-effective way to communicate is to disseminate information on their websites, so the contents must be culturally and cognitively friendly to the target readers. What's more, the processes of research and development for coronary stents are time-consuming and highly technical, so publishing news is almost a routine task for medical device companies, especially for those listed in Table 6-1. It is in this context that coronary stent news has a key role to play.

6.3　Modal Verbs in Discourses

The unique language phenomenon of modal verbs is the locus of cognitive grammar studies. At the semantic level, they have been discussed with the grounding theory from their meaning conceptualization processes to explore how the conceptions of physical or abstract force in modal verbs are reflected in discoursal structures, with various linguistic choices and modal forms.

6.3.1　Modal verbs and their studies

Modal verbs are the most important way of expressing modality meaning. From the semantic view, Lyons (1977: 452) defines that "modality is a means used by a speaker to express his opinion or attitude towards the proposition that the sentence expresses or the situation that the proposition describes". In this sense, modality meaning can be expressed in many forms, including adjectives like "probable", nouns like "probability", adverbs like "probably" and verbs like "will". Perkins (1983) suggests modality as the conceptual context in which an event or proposition is established or not, that is, the so-called possible world. He added quasi-auxiliary modal expressions (such as "have to"), modal nominal expressions (such as "assertion"), modal lexical verbs (such as "order"), if clauses, and interrogative sentences, etc. Quirk et al. (1985) propose modality as the restrictive element of a sentence, which reflects the speaker's judgment on the possibility of a proposition. Palmer (2001) notes that modality is the grammaticalization of the speaker's subjective attitudes and opinions and is concerned with the status of the proposition that describes the event. From the perspective of SFL, Halliday and Matthiessen (2004) argue that modality is an important part of interpersonal meta-function and defines modality as the range of likelihood lying between positive polarity (yes) and negative polarity (no). The realization of modality meaning covers a wider range of forms including modal verbs, modal adjuncts, the combination of modal verbs and modal adjuncts, and interpersonal metaphors. Therefore, it can be concluded that modality is associated with notions such as possibility or necessity, propositional attitudes, and speakers' attitudes. The present research adopts Palmer's (2001) definition as a working definition that modality is the speaker's subjective attitude towards the truth value of a proposition or the reality of an event. On the one hand, it emphasizes that a sentence consists of a proposition and the speaker's subjectivity. On the other hand, the truth value or the potentiality of a proposition is stated. Therefore, when a proposition (true or false) is restricted by a restrictive element to express modality, the restrictive element is regarded as a modal marker.

For epistemic modality, Lyons (1977: 797) sees epistemic modality as "any utterance in which the speaker explicitly qualifies his commitment to the truth of the proposition expressed by the sentence he utters". As Coates (1985: 18) sees it, epistemic modality concerns with "the speaker's assumptions, or assessment of possibilities, and in most cases, it indicates the speaker's confidence or lack of confidence in the truth of the proposition expressed". There are three types of judgment in the category of epistemic modality. Speculative modality means uncertainty; deductive modality indicates an inference from observable evidence; assumptive modality indicates an inference from what is generally known. For deontic modality, it concerns the necessity or possibility of acts in view of social rules or values, which means that the act is pressed by morally responsible agents (Lyons 1977). It is essentially obligative, permissive and commissive. A speaker using deontic modals can give permission ("may/can"), lay an obligation ("must"), or make a promise or threat ("shall") (Palmer 1990). For dynamic modality, it is concerned with ability and willingness rather than speaker's attitude or opinion, which are expressed by the modal verbs "can" and "will" in English. Palmer (1990) argues that the difference between dynamic and deontic modality is the notion of control which means the controller of the event. With dynamic modality, the control is internal to the subject. By contrast, the deontic modality indicates that the event is controlled by external circumstances.

In SFL, language is conceived as a resource for making meanings. Through mood and modality, Halliday (1994) proposes that interpersonal meta-function is reflected in the status, attitude, and motivation of the speaker and his evaluation of things. A lot of studies on modal verbs mainly discussed their function in various discourses, media discourses (Liu 2008; Ren & Wang 2017; Yang et al. 2017), academic discourses (Li 2001; Halliday 1994), legal discourses (Ma et al. 2017), and others. Liu (2008) finds that modal verbs in media discourses are important in establishing an objective and reliable tone, realizing interpersonal meaning in discourses. Ren and Wang (2017) comparatively analyse the Chinese and English modality systems in terms of their modal orientation, modal values and modal types and revealed that English political news discourses prefer to use more modals indicating probability and inclination while Chinese political news discourses favour those indicating obligation and inclination. Li (2001) argues that epistemic modality is a typical feature of speakers' efforts to pursue objectivity in academic discourses, which makes information more acceptable to readers. Investigating the value distribution of epistemic modality, their orientation, and functions in medical discourses, Yang et al. (2017) consider that the use of low and median value, and explicitly subjective and objective orientations of modal expressions contributes to making tentative, reserved, and objective claims. Modal expressions, such as modal verbs, can reveal and reflect speakers' different stances, statues and power, which powerfully help addressers realize regulation, permission, authorization, and prohibition, whereas it is detrimental to the credibility and accuracy of the statements of addressees. Vergaro (2004: 185), in sales promotional letters, deems that mood and modality can have an addressee-oriented function especially when they are used for the expression of politeness. No matter what discourses the modal verbs are used in, they prove functional in interpersonal meaning and to some extent reflect the characteristics and uniqueness of the discourses.

6.3.2 Classification of modal verbs

Researchers have made considerable attempts in classifying modality from different perspectives and based on different criteria. For instance, Coates (1985) groups modality into root and epistemic modality. Halliday and Matthiessen (2004) classifies modality into modalization and modulation. Bybee et al. (1994) and Bybee and Fleischman (1995) distinguish between agent-oriented modality and epistemic modality. Since the author applies cross-linguistic comparison study, she uses Palmer's classification as he has provided evidence for the cross-language studies of modalities and modal systems. In addition, Chinese and English in the grammatical category of modality have a strong commonality because they both use modal verbs as the main means of modality expression (Zhu 2005). Employing a typological approach, Palmer (2001: 22) divides modality into propositional and event modality shown in Figure 6-1. The former describes a speaker's attitude to the status of a proposition while the latter refers to events that are not actualized.

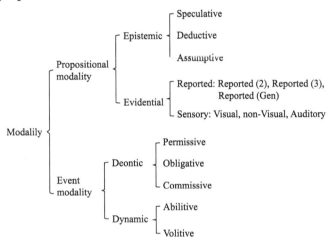

Figure 6-1   The classification of modality system (Palmer 2001: 22)

To make it focused, this research only focuses on modal verbs which is the core of modality system particularly in English. Quirk et al. (1985: 137) suggest central modals verbs cover "can, could, may, might, will, would, shall, should, must" and so on, and marginal modal verbs cover "dare, need, ought to, used to" and so on. Peng (2007) holds that prototypical Chinese modal verbs are "能(够)(can)", "要(will/should)", "会(will/can)", "应该(应当)(should)", "(可)(can)", "肯(be willing to)", "敢(dare)", "得(děi)(have to)", "该(should)", "可能 (may)", "想(be willing to)", "一定(must)", "准(allow)" and non-prototypical Chinese modal verbs are "必须(must)", "肯定(must)", "乐意/情愿/愿意(be willing to)", "许(allow)". This chapter only covers nine central English modal verbs and thirteen central Chinese modal verbs. The polysemic modals are illustrated with examples from Coates (1985) and Palmer (1990), and Peng (2007) and Zhu (2005). The result of the classification is summarized in Table 6-2.

Table 6-2 The classification of English and Chinese central modal verbs

Modality	Semantic meaning	English Modal verbs	Chinese Modal verbs
Epistemic modality	speculative	may, might, could	可能(may), 能(够)(could)
	deductive	must, should	必然(must), 一定(must), 肯定(must), 得(have to), 要(will), 准(allow)
	assumptive	will, would	会(will), 应该(应当/该/应/当)(should)
Deontic modality	permissive	may, can, could, might	能(够)(can), 可(以) (may), 许(allow), 准(allow)
	obligative	must, should, ought to	必须(must), 应该(should), 得(have to), 要(must)
	commissive	shall, will	会(may), 肯定(must), 一定(must), 准(allow)
Dynamic modality	ablitive	can, could	可以(can), 会(can), 能(够)(can)
	volitive	will, shall, would	要(will), 肯(想/愿意)(be willing to)
	courage	dare	敢(dare)

English modal verbs studied here are as follows.

1. Must

Deontic meaning (obligation)

> You <u>must</u> play this ten times over. (Coates 1985: 31)

Epistemic meaning (necessity)

> That place <u>must</u> make quite a profit for it was packed out and has been all week. (Coates 1985: 31)

2. May/might

Epistemic meaning (possibility)

> You <u>may</u> not like the idea of it, but let me explain. (Palmer 1990: 51)
> You think someone <u>might</u> be watching us. (Palmer 1990: 58)

Deontic meaning (permission)

> If you want to recall the doctor, you <u>may</u> do so. (Palmer 1990: 71)
> I said he <u>might</u> come tomorrow. (Palmer 1990: 43)

3. Will
Epistemic meaning (probability)

John <u>will</u> be in his office. (Palmer 1990: 57)

Dynamic meaning (volition)

Give them the name of someone who <u>will</u> sign for it and take it in if you are not at home. (Coates 1985: 171)

4. Can
Deontic meaning (Permission)

You <u>can</u> go into the bathroom. (Coates 1985: 87)

Dynamic meaning (ability/possibility)

I <u>can</u> only type very slowly as I am quite a beginner. (Coates 1985: 89)
Signs are the only things you <u>can</u> observe. (Palmer 1990: 83)

5. Could
Epistemic meaning (possibility)

I <u>could</u> get held up for anything up to a week. (Coates 1985: 108)

Dynamic meaning (past of can: ability/possibility)

I <u>could</u> just touch the roof. (Coates 1985: 111)
We <u>could</u> have another holiday. (Coates 1985: 108)

Deontic meaning (permission)

They <u>could</u> do quite legally. (Coates 1985: 108)

6. Should
Deontic meaning (obligation)

You <u>should</u> walk round the ramparts of the old city too. (Coates 1985: 58)

Epistemic meaning (necessity)

The trip <u>should</u> take about sixteen days. (Coates 1985: 64)

7. Would
Epistemic meaning (probability: predictability/prediction)

They <u>would</u> both go away holding to their own views. (Coates 1985: 205)
Mary was waiting to see what <u>would</u> happen. (Coates 1985: 205)

Dynamic meaning (past of will: volition)

I <u>would</u> take an appointment there. (Coates 1985: 205)

8. Shall
Deontic meaning (commitment)

He <u>shall</u> be there by six. (Palmer 1990: 74)

Dynamic meaning (volition)

I <u>shall</u> always be grateful. (Coates 1985: 195)

Chinese modal verbs studied here are as follows.

1. 能(够)(can)
Deontic meaning (Permission)

我<u>能</u>走了吗? (Peng 2007: 151)
(<u>Can</u> I go?)

Dynamic meaning (ability/possibility)

他<u>能</u>听懂英语了。(Peng 2007: 148)
(He <u>can</u> understand English.)
从广州两小时就<u>能</u>到韶关。
(You <u>can</u> get to Shaoguan from Guangzhou in two hours.)

2. 要(will/should)
Epistemic meaning (necessity)

那是很野蛮的运动，<u>要</u>伤身体的。(Peng 2007: 139)
(It's a very savage sport, it <u>will</u> hurt your body.)

Deontic meaning (obligation)

路有些远，男同学<u>要</u>帮着女同学。(Peng 2007: 138)

(It is far, and the boys <u>should</u> help the girls.)

Dynamic meaning (volition)

我不在你们这儿上学了，我<u>要</u>回去。(Peng 2007: 137)

(I'm not going to school with you anymore, and I <u>will</u> be back.)

3. 会(will/can)

Epistemic meaning (probability)

现在他不<u>会</u>在家里。(Peng 2007: 144)

(Now he <u>will</u> not be at home.)

Deontic meaning (commitment)

我<u>会</u>保护你。(Peng 2007: 143)

(I <u>will</u> protect you.)

Dynamic meaning (ability)

以前他不怎么<u>会</u>说普通话，现在会(说)了。(Peng 2007: 141)

(He wouldn't speak Mandarin very much before, now he <u>can</u>.)

4. 应该(应当/该) (should)

Epistemic meaning (probability)

他昨天动身的,今天<u>应该</u>到了。(Peng 2007: 145)

(He left yesterday, and he <u>should</u> be here today.)

Deontic meaning (obligation)

你<u>应该</u>去！(Peng 2007: 145)

(You <u>should</u> go!)

5. 可(以) (can)

Deontic meaning (permission)

你可以回去了。(Peng 2007: 157)

(You can go back.)

Dynamic meaning (ability)

我可以控制。(Peng 2007: 154)

(I can control it.)

6. 得(děi) (have to)

Epistemic meaning (deduction)

他准得来。(Peng 2007: 130)

(He has to come.)

Deontic meaning (obligation)

这件事得你来做。(Peng 2007: 130)

(You have to do that.)

7. 一定(must)

Epistemic meaning (necessity)

他一定要去，就让他去吧。(Peng 2007: 133)

(If he must go, let him go.)

Deontic meaning (obligation)

你一定别忘了。(Peng 2007: 133)

(You must not forget it.)

8. 准 (must/allow)

Epistemic meaning (necessity)

人跑不了，准在这院里。(Peng 2007: 136)

(They can't run away, and they must be in this courtyard.)

Deontic meaning (permission)

你不准进这三间房。(Peng 2007: 137)

(You are not <u>allowed</u> to enter the three rooms.)

Modal verb as a language resource concerns the speaker's assessment of, and subjective attitude towards the truth value of a proposition or the potentiality of an event. It is well considered as an objective communication tool and an essential discursive strategy involving interpersonal meaning to express tentativeness, uncertainty, negotiation etc. (e.g. Yang et al. 2016). Based on the categories of modal verbs and their applications in grounding contexts, the author analyses them within the context of promotional discourses of medical devices in both Chinese and English texts.

6.4　Modal Verbs in Promotional Discourses of MDPNs

Cognitive linguists uphold that meaning is constructed through conceptualization. This part is to analyse the conceptualization of modal verbs, uncovering the expressions of the source, or the locus of the potency, with a target of the directed potency and an agent who acts in hopes of revealing substantial differences in the nature of modals conceptual structure reflected in the authentic texts.

6.4.1　Modal grounding analysis of English discourses

Table 6-3 shows the meaning distribution of English modals. Within epistemic modality, possibility, probability, and necessity are distinguished as a proposition which is considered to be uncertain, probable or be based on certain judgements. Within dynamic modality, ability and neutral possibility are distinguished as the meaning of "can" which extends "from the core of 'ability' to the periphery of 'possibility'" (Coates 1985). Within deontic modality, only obligation is involved. Of the 17 531 English words, modal verbs appeared 139 times, accounting for about 0.79%. It means that the frequency of modal verbs in English MDPNs is 79 times per 10,000 words.

Table 6-3   Meaning distribution of English modal verbs

Modal verbs	Epistemic modality			Dynamic modality		Deontic modality	Total
	Possibility	Probability	Necessity	Ability	Neutral possibility	Obligation	
will	0	50	0	0	0	0	50 (35.97%)
can	0	0	0	28	13	0	41 (29.50%)
may	33	0	0	0	0	0	33 (23.74%)
could	7	0	0	0	0	0	7 (5.04%)
should	0	0	1	0	0	2	3 (2.16%)
might	3	0	0	0	0	0	3 (2.16%)
would	0	2	0	0	0	0	2 (1.44%)
Total	96 (69.06%)			41 (29.50%)		2 (1.44%)	139 (100.00%)

On the whole, it reveals that the three modalities follow the pattern: epistemic modality appears most frequently, dynamic modality ranks the second place and deontic modality ranks the third. For specific modals, "will" is used most, followed by "can", "may" and "could". Barely used are "should" , "might" and "would". They are analysed according to their importance and typicality.

6.4.1.1　Epistemic "will"

"Will" is a kind of epistemic marker and it is justified to express a reasonable conclusion as the speaker always makes a claim based on repeated experiences and common sense (Palmer 1990). The conceptual construal of epistemic "will" originates from one's desire and intention (Bybee et al. 1994). Therefore, epistemic "will" can be used to make predictions that are planned, and envisaged.

Epistemic "will" appeared most frequently in the English discourses studied, indicating that English producers quite frequently make future predictions. On the one hand, since medical companies need to issue the latest findings and research results as soon as possible and many other studies or research will be carried out in the future, prediction is undoubtedly favoured by promotional news discourses in the medical fields. On the other hand, it also conveys a high degree of writers' confidence in the truth value of the proposition based on evidence and knowledge of the present or past situation and it is quite common in science. It is illustrated in the following examples.

Example 32 (Source: ET13)

We hope these data **will** support our submission to the FDA for a one-month DAPT indication for high-bleeding risk patients treated with Resolute Onyx. (Medtronic Onyx ONE Clear Study of One-Month Dual-Antiplatelet Therapy in High Bleeding Risk Stent Patients Beats Performance Goal, Medtronic, 30 April, 2020)[1]

Example 33 (Source: ET2)

We believe the results from DAPT-STEMI, in addition to the future outcomes from the RESOLUTE ONYX ONE study, **will** help to inform DAPT guidelines for newer-generation DES. (Independent Study Shows New Data on Shortened DAPT in STEMI Patients with Medtronic Resolute Integrity Drug-Eluting Stent, Medtronic. November 1, 2017)[2]

Instead of driving the profiled process, epistemic "will" mainly reflects the writers' efforts in assessing the likelihood of a proposition based on external evidences. The potency of the conceptualizer inheres in the ground, consisting of the conceptualizer's knowledge and experience. In these two examples demonstrated in Figure 6-2(a), the conceptualizer "we" in Examples 32 and 33 is in the maximal scope, becoming the marginal focus. The involvement of the ground can increase the subjectivity of the proposition. Inference evidence such as "these data" and "the results" is clearly stated and profiled in the IS scope. Therefore, the evidence and the events are right on the focus of readers' attention. We can conclude that the modal meaning of prediction about the

---

① https://news.medtronic.com/2020-03-30-Medtronic-Onyx-ONE-Clear-Study-of-One-Month-Dual-Antiplatelet-Therapy-in-High-Bleeding-Risk-Stent-Patients-Beats-Performance-Goal

② https://news.medtronic.com/2017-11-01-Independent-Study-Shows-New-Data-on-Shortened-DAPT-in-STEMI-Patients- with-Medtronic-Resolute-Integrity-Drug-Eluting-Stent

projected future events is mainly made based on discourse producers' existing knowledge of and confidence in the scientific results and experimental data, strengthening Americans' scientific spirit and truth-seeking cultural background and thus conforming to readers' preferences. At the same time, the involvement of discourse producers on the ground increases the subjectivity of the texts.

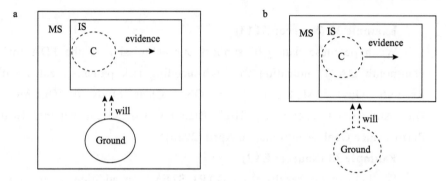

Figure 6-2   Conceptual construal of epistemic "will"

Example 34 (Source: ET17)

Abbott's new OCT virtual reality-based training programs, **will** dramatically enhance decision-making for physicians who utilize OCT instead of angiography. (ABBOTT Launches First Optical Coherence Tomography Virtual Reality Training Program for Cardiologists. 9 December, 2020)[①]

The repeated experience and common sense can also be conveyed through epistemic "will" in Example 34. As shown in Figure 6-2(b), the conceptualizer is not mentioned. The ground is off the stage, which is subjectively construed and thus the prediction wins the maximal objectivity. The profiled process and inference evidence of "reality-based training programs" are clearly stated and profiled onstage. "Reality-based training programs" serves as an index pointing towards a fact-oriented approach. Together, these elements contribute to a collective understanding, facilitating access for patients to coronary stents that

---

① https://abbott.mediaroom.com/2020-12-09-Abbott-Launches-First-Optical-Coherence-Tomography-Virtual-Reality- Training-Program-for-Cardiologists

are not only of superior quality but also incorporate the latest technological innovations. Patients, thus, can have access to coronary stents with better quality and new technology. The discourse producers make an assessment of the possibility of the proposition objectively which equals to a fact. Thus, "will" expresses a high degree of confidence towards the proposition because it is true in discourse producers' reality. Whether the ground is involved or not, the discourse producers use epistemic "will" to express envisaged or planned events.

6.4.1.2   Dynamic "can"

The modal verb "can" has dynamic meanings in contexts. Generally, it has two main forces, which is labelled as "can1" and "can2". "can1" refers to the ability of the participant's internal enabling conditions, indicating the source, target and agent of the modal force. They identically refer to the trajector whose typical grammatical expression is the clausal subject. Apart from the internal enabling conditions, the dynamic "can2" represents external possibility resulting from circumstantial conditions in which an event is possible. The few cases in discourses all concern the topic of emergent circumstances caused by changes in coronary vessels. Similarly, shown in Figure 6-3(a), the force implementation process is onstage, objectively construed.

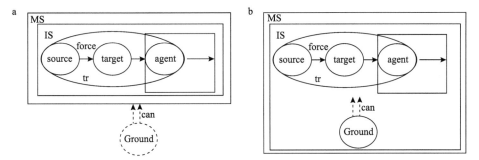

Figure 6-3   Conceptual construal of dynamic "can"

Example 35 (Source: ET19)

The XIENCE stent is used in life-saving treatments that **can1** help prevent or treat heart attacks and has now consistently been proven safe with short DAPT strategies for HBR patients. (Abbott's XIENCE™ Stent Receives European Approval for One-Month Dual Anti-Platelet Therapy (DAPT) for High Bleeding Risk Patients, Abbott Laboratories, April 6, 2021)[①]

Example 36 (Source: ET29)

By adding these new products to our portfolio, we **can2** make the most significant contribution to the healthcare system and deliver innovative products and solutions that our customers and their patients are seeking. (Cordis Showcases Comprehensive Interventional Cardiology Portfolio with Coronary Stents at TCT, Cardinal Health, October, 30,2017)[②]

In Example 35, "can1" in dynamic modality indicates ability, while in Example 36, "can2" in dynamic modality indicates neutral possibility. It is quite understandable to see many modal verbs of dynamic "can1" employed in medical discourses. Apart from the goal of boasting excellent features of the stents available or newly approved, another goal aims to distinguish the company from other medical device companies by displaying its innovative capabilities.

The force implementation process of modal force and the profiled events are onstage sketched in Figure 6-3. The role of the source, target, and agent of the modal force is identical, and it refers to the trajector whose typical grammatical expression is the clausal subject. The source of the modal force comes from the innate feature of the subject for the occurrence of the event. The force is indicated by the bold arrow. The agent of the action indicates that the subject is able to act. In Example 35, no ground information is mentioned and thus the ground is offstage shown in Figure 6-3(a), with the onstage elements objectively construed. The subject "XIENCE stent" indicates that the internal feature of the stent gives itself the modal force and carries out the potential action. In Example 36 shown in Figure 6-3(b), subject "we", indicates that workers in the medical device company Cordis are capable of making a difference in the healthcare industry. However, it is onstage in the IS scope, representing a subjective construal towards the action as the ground

---

① https://abbott.mediaroom.com/2021-04-06-Abbotts-XIENCE-TM-Stent-Receives-European-Approval-for-One-Month-Dual-Anti-Platelet-Therapy-DAPT-for-High-Bleeding-Risk-Patients

② https://newsroom.cardinalhealth.com/company-news?item=123137

information got involved in the communication. The ability of the products and company onstage are highlighted with maximal salience. So examples of "can1" highlight features that are specific and available to the company or the product being referred to, thus building a favourable company image and strong product brand.

Example 37 (Source: ET1)

Treatment of the left main coronary artery is critical as the artery supplies the majority of blood to the left side of the heart; a narrowing in this vessel **can2** place the patient at high risk for life-threatening events. (Medtronic Adds New Resolute Onyx(TM) Drug-Eluting Stent Sizes and Expands Indications, TCTMD, 1 February, 2016) [1]

In Example 37, the subject "a narrowing in this vessel" is a circumstance, imposing a modal force on the target. The enabling condition makes it possible for the agent to perform the potential act. The dynamic "can2" activates the potency of the circumstances to make something happen in an objective way.

6.4.1.3　Epistemic "may"

As stated in epistemic "will", epistemic modality concerns the speakers' assessment of the strength of modal force. The strength of speaker's belief conveyed by "may" is lower than that of epistemic "will". It can be interpreted as a possible conclusion made by the speaker.

Example 38 (Source: ET 8)

These data help expand the growing body of clinical evidence that **may** support physicians in tailoring DAPT regimens for complex patients. (Independent Stent Imaging Study Shows Excellent Healing Profile with Resolute Onyx DES in Complex Patients with Coronary Artery Disease, Medtronic, May 24, 2018)[2]

---

[1] https://www.tctmd.com/news/medtronic-adds-new-resolute-onyxtm-drug-eluting-stent-sizes-and-expands-indications

[2] https://news.medtronic.com/2018-05-24-Independent-Stent-Imaging-Study-Shows-Excellent-Healing-Profile-with- Resolute-Onyx-DES-in-Complex-Patients-with-Coronary-Artery-Disease

Example 39 (Source: ET15)

Data from these late-breaking trials **may** help physicians rethink what is possible in managing patients with coronary artery disease and heart failure. (Late Breaking Data Presentations at ACC 2019 Highlight Abbott's Leading Cardiovascular Portfolio, Abbott Laboratories, March 6, 2019)[①]

In promotional news discourses of the medical fields, the application of "may" is essential to avoid absoluteness and leave readers room for action. Here, the conceptualization of modal "may" is sketched in Figure 6-4.

The conceptualizer (C) in Figure 6-4 is not stated in the sentence, and thus is circled by dotted line. In Examples 38 and 39, "clinical evidence" and "data from these late-breaking trials" are put onstage by the producers who believe that they are the most convincing scientific evidences. It is this evidence that boosts discourse producers' confidence in reasoning possible events. The epistemic use of modal verb "may" in English discourses reflects the possibility of the potential acts based on the discourse producers' knowledge of the clinical data.

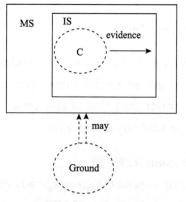

Figure 6-4　Conceptual construal of epistemic "may"

6.4.1.4　Epistemic "could"

As suggested by Palmer (1987) on the classification of modal verbs, the modal verb "could" can also be used to imply a possible conclusion based on

---

① https://abbott.mediaroom.com/2019-03-06-Late-Breaking-Data-Presentations-at-ACC-2019-Highlight-Abbotts-Leading- Cardiovascular-Portfolio

knowing facts. It is typically associated with a weak epistemic judgment. In addition, modal verb "could" symbolizes a kind of euphemism and indirectness, leaving room for interpersonal negotiation.

Example 40 (Source: ET4)

The ZEUS trial and subsequently, the LEADERS-FREE trial (which evaluated a different DCS vs. BMS), showed that other DES systems **could** be a better alternative to BMS in patients with a high risk of bleeding. (Medtronic Announces Randomized Global Resolute Onyx(TM) DES One-Month Dual Antiplatelet Therapy Study to Address Critical Unanswered Question in Interventional Cardiology, Medtronic, August 2017)[①]

Epistemic "could" in English MDPNs is employed to convey negotiation and tentativeness. Coates (1985) notes that epistemic "could" is very similar to epistemic "may", thus sharing the same conceptualization process shown in Figure 6-5.

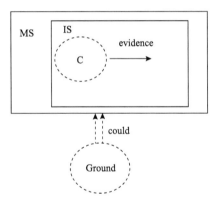

Figure 6-5   Conceptual construal of epistemic "could"

In Figure 6-5, the degree of modal force relies on solid evidence. The source modal force comes from the solid evidence "the ZEUS trial and subsequently, the LEADERS-FREE trial" in Example 40. Although there are convincing trials to prove the possibility of the profiled events, the English discourse producers still express uncertainty in reasoning to show their

---

① https://news.medtronic.com/2017-08-14-Medtronic-Announces-Randomized-Global-Resolute-Onyx-TM-DES-One-Month-Dual-Antiplatelet-Therapy-Study-to-Address-Critical-Unanswered-Question-in-Interventional-Cardiology. ZEUS means "Zettawatt-Equivalent Ultrashort pulse laser System".

skepticism about the utterance, indicating their prudence.

6.4.2　Modal grounding analysis of Chinese discourses

Table 6-4 shows the meaning distribution of Chinese modal verbs. The negative forms can be spotted in the Chinese discourses but only in a few cases with "不会(won't)". For epistemic modality, possibility, probability, and necessity are detected. Within dynamic modality, ability and volition are distinguished as the meaning extends from ability to willingness. Within deontic modality, only obligation is involved. Of the 43,098 Chinese characters, modal verbs appeared 116 times, accounting for about 0.27%. It means that the frequency of modal verbs in Chinese discourses is about 27 times per 10,000 characters.

Table 6-4　Meaning distribution of Chinese modal verbs

Modal verbs	Epistemic modality			Dynamic modality		Deontic modality	Total
	Possibility	Probability	Necessity	Ability	Volition	Obligation	
能(够)(can)	0	0	0	50	0	0	50(43.10%)
可(以)(can)	0	0	0	31	0	0	31(26.72%)
会(will) 不会(won't)	0	11 6	0	0	0	0	17(14.66%)
可能(may)	7	0	0	0	0	0	7(6.03%)
要(will/should)	0	1	0	0	1	2	4(3.45%)
(应)该(should)	0	0	0	0	0	3	3(2.59%)
一定(must)	0	0	2	0	0	0	2(1.72%)
想(be willing to)	0	0	0	0	1	0	1(0.86%)
敢(dare)	0	0	0	0	1	0	1(0.86%)
Total	27(23.28%)			84(72.41%)		5(4.31%)	116(100%)

Accordingly, it reveals that the three modalities follow the pattern: dynamic modality ranks at the top, epistemic modality ranks second, and deontic modality ranks third. For specific modals, the variety of Chinese modal verbs is more diverse than English ones, but they display different degrees of preference. "能(够)(can)" is used most, followed by "可(以)(can)", "会(will)/不会(won't)" and "可能(may)". Correspondingly, this part only goes through the top four occurrence modals "能(够)(can)", "可(以)(can)", "会(will)", and "可能(may)".

6.4.2.1　Dynamic "能(够)(can)"

"能(够)(can)" conveys epistemic, dynamic, and deontic meanings. All cases found in Chinese MDPNs are dynamically used to express subject-oriented ability. Peng (2007) clarifies that dynamic ability typically relates to the ability or conditions to do something or a certain use/function. Medical device companies prefer to use "能(够)(can)" to demonstrate their innovative capabilities and their products' excellent qualities.

Example 41 (Source: CT27)

这一涂层**能够**加速内膜覆盖速度，促进内膜的功能性愈合，同时还**能够**减少涂层下金属支架中重金属离子的释放。(PIONEER III 研究结果正式发表——中国原创愈合导向药物洗脱支架安全有效性获得验证,赛诺医疗, 2021 年 4 月 29 日)①

This coating **can** accelerate the coverage rate of intima, promote the functional healing of intima, and **can** also reduce the release of heavy metal ions in the metal scaffold under the coating. (PIONEER III research results are officially published—Chinese original healing-oriented drug-eluting stent has been verified for safety and effectiveness, SINOMED, 29 April, 2021)

Example 42 (Source: CT30)

"使用 NeoVas 支架，**能换来** 3 年以后自由自在的生命与生活，这种自由是无价的。"（NeoVas 诞生记：乐普医疗 20 年创新的中国担当, 乐普医疗, 2019 年 4 月 2 日）②

"Using NeoVas stent **can exchange** free life in three years. This

---

① http://www.sinomed.com/zh-hans/2021/04/29/copy-of
② https://www.lepumedical.com/newList.html

freedom is priceless." (The birth of NeoVas: Lepu Medical's 20-year innovation in China MicroPort Medical, Lepu Medical, 2 April, 2019)

Example 43 (Source: CT30)

我们研发支架的过程有成功，也有失败，有过不同水平的尝试和长期坚持的努力，这才**能够**实现从跟跑到领跑，从仿制到创新的跨越。（NeoVas 诞生记：乐普医疗 20 年创新的中国担当,乐普医疗，2019 年 4 月 2 日）①

We have both succeeded and failed in the process of stent R&D. We have tried at different levels and made long-term efforts. Only in this way **can** we realize the leap from following to leading, from imitation to innovation. (The birth of NeoVas: Lepu Medical's 20-year innovation in China MicroPort Medical, Lepu Medical, 2 April, 2019)

The product's functional ability, the animate participant's internal ability and conditional ability are widely presented in discourses. It is the modal force that activates the subject to realize its internal features for the occurrence of the event. The force implementation process and the profiled process are all onstage, realizing objective construal. The source, target and agent of the modal force are the same, played by the clausal subject. In Example 41, the source of force comes from the subject "这一涂层(this coating)" which has some inherent properties to send an internal force to itself and forces the agent to carry out the potential acts. The subject "使用 NeoVas 支架(using NeoVas stent)" in Example 42 as a circumstance makes it possible for patients to live a free life. These two examples do not mention the conceptualizer as seen in Figure 6-6(a), so the potential acts are objectively construed. In Example 43, the source of the modal force comes from the animate subject "我们(we)" highlighted in IS scope, realizing maximal subjectivity seen in Figure 6-6(b). It is the mental ability that imposes force on the target and allows the agent to carry out the act. We can conclude that dynamic "能(够)(can)" in Chinese MDPNs objectively construes the function of stents but subjectively construes stents' excellent performances.

---

① https://www.lepumedical.com/newList.html

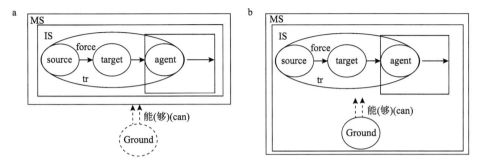

Figure 6-6 Conceptual construal of dynamic "能(够)(can)"

6.4.2.2 Dynamic "可(以)(can)"

According to Peng (2007: 152-158), the dynamic ability of "可(以) (can)" involves three aspects like "能(够) (can)": the ability or conditions to do something or a certain use/function. In this sense, the dynamic meaning of "能(够) (can)" and "可 (以) (can)" is almost the same. This chapter confirms that subject-oriented ability is often realized by modal verbs "能(够) (can)" and "可(以) (can)". All cases are used to express dynamic ability in the Chinese MDPNs.

Example 44 (Source: CT24)

中国原创的产品也**可以**帮助建立新的技术标准，中国原创力量也**可以**推动心血管介入治疗领域的技术发展。（我国自主研发药物洗脱支架获得欧洲 CE 批准，赛诺医疗/搜狐网，2019 年 12 月 23 日）①

China's original products **can** also help establish new technical standards and **can** also promote the technical development of cardiovascular interventional therapy. (Drug eluting stents independently developed in China have been approved by European CE, SINOMED / Sohu.com, 23 December, 2019)

Example 45 (Source: CT24)

赛诺医疗产品成功进入国际发达市场，标志着中国自主研发高端医疗器械**可以**不断突破技术壁垒。(我国自主研发药物洗脱支架获得欧洲 CE 批准，赛诺医疗/搜狐网，2019 年 12 月 23 日）②

---

① https://www.sohu.com/a/362247276_186367
② https://www.sohu.com/a/362247276_186367

The successful entry of SINOMED products into the internationally developed markets indicates that China's independent research and development of high-end medical devices **can** break through technical barriers. (Drug eluting stents independently developed in China have been approved by European CE, SINOMED/ Sohu.com, 23 December, 2019)

The locus of the potency tends to be the clausal subject which is activated by the dynamic "可(以) (can)". Its conceptual construal process is sketched in Figure 6-7.

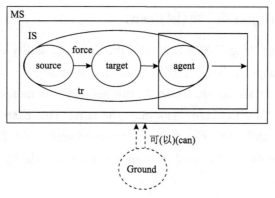

Figure 6-7 Conceptual construal of dynamic "可(以)(can)"

In Example 44, the subject "中国原创的产品 (China's original products)" has the inner source of strength which is continuous and dynamic. This inner force forces itself to carry out actions that are innovative and technically competitive. In Example 45, the modal force comes from the clausal subject "中国自主研发高端医疗器械 (China's independent research and development of high-end medical devices)". It is the same as what has been discussed in Example 43, emphasizing the capabilities of Chinese companies themselves. The subject imposes the force on itself and then enables the agent itself to carry out the act. The source, target and agent of the modal force are identical and are put onstage for objective construal. We can see that the use of "可(以) (can)" regards products created in China as the trajector and highlights the technological innovations objectively.

6.4.2.3　Epistemic "会(will)"

"会(will)" can be used to express epistemic, deontic, and dynamic modality, but the cases identified are all epistemically used. For epistemic meaning, "会(will)" indicates probability, a reasonable inference (Peng 2007: 83). Some scholars believe that "会(will)" has a high degree of possibility (Peng 2007). It can be found in future tense. In this chapter, epistemic "会 (will)" mainly focuses on the probability of products' excellent performance.

> **Example 46 (Source: CT27)**
> Leon 教授进一步解释, HT-DES 在植入后第一个月就**会**完成至少 80% 的药物释放。(PIONEER III 研究结果正式发表——中国原创愈合导向药物洗脱支架安全有效性获得验证, 赛诺医疗, 2021 年 4 月 29)[①]
>
> Professor Leon further explained that HT-DES **will** release at least 80% of the drug in the first month after implantation. (PIONEER III research results are officially published—Chinese original healing-oriented drug-eluting stent has been verified for safety and effectiveness, SINOMED, 29 April, 2021)
>
> **Example 47 (Source: CT22)**
> 我们相信产品一经上市, 将**会**在东亚地区造福更多患者。(蓝帆医疗新一代 Biofreedom™ Ultra 钴铬合金支架在韩国、泰国获批, 蓝帆医疗, 2021 年 3 月 3 日)[②]
>
> We believe that once the product is launched, it **will** benefit more patients in East Asia. （Bluesail medical' new generation Biofreedom™ Ultra cobalt chromium alloy support was approved in Republic of Korea and Thailand，Bluesail Medical, 3 March, 2021）

"会 (will)" does not intend to affect a potential process, but makes a prediction based on the speaker's assessment of the normal course of events for the future (known reality) and his knowledge of the unknown reality (See Figure 6-8).

[①] http://www.sinomed.com/zh-hans/2021/04/29/copy-of

[②] https://www.bluesail.cn/en/enterpriseinformation/1766.htm

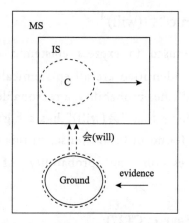

Figure 6-8 Conceptual construal of epistemic "会(will)"

As shown in Figure 6-8, modal force comes from the ground based on Professor Leon's explanation (see Example 46) which is cited as evidence to enhance the persuasiveness of the proposition. Often experts' explanations represent authority and accuracy and thus the proposition is highly possible. "我们 (we)" in Example 47 is stated in the sentence, thus surrounded by a solid line in maximal scope (MS) shown in Figure 6-8. The evidence might lie in conceptualizer's encyclopaedia knowledge about the regular process of a listed product. We can conclude that Chinese discourse producers prefer to employ "会 (will)" to predict an envisaged future by highlighting experts' authority and their own experience, instead of convincing data as English discourse producers do. Epistemic use of "会 (will)" often combines with different degrees of subjectivity seen from the construal process.

6.4.2.4 Epistemic "可能(may)"

As Peng (2007) deems, modal verb "可能 (may)" is univocal, and specializes in cognitive possibility. The weak form of modal verb "可能 (may)" is univocal and specialized in epistemic possibility.

Example 48 (Source: CT2)
Firesorb™（火鹮）较薄的支架壁厚度使产品的通过外径得以减少，并**可能**缩短降解时间，有效降低血栓形成的风险。(业内第二代生物全可吸收血管支架系统 Firesorb™（火鹮）通过 CFDA 创新医疗器械特别审批

申请, 微创, 2016 年 6 月 13 日)①

The thinner wall of Firesorb™ reduces the crossing profile of the product, and **may** shorten the degradation time, effectively reducing the risk of thrombosis. (The industry's second-generation biological fully absorbable vascular stent system Firesorb™ has passed the special approval application for CFDA (China Food and Drug Administration) innovative medical devices, MicroPort, June 13, 2016)

It is quite understandable that news discourses may use the epistemic modal verbs to express uncertainty, especially in the technology fields. The construal process of modal verb "可能 (may)" is sketched in Figure 6-9, similar to the English epistemic "may".

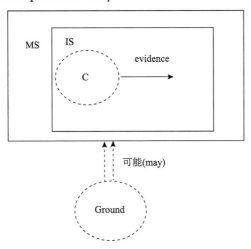

Figure 6-9 Conceptual construal of epistemic "可能(may)"

The ground is offstage and only the proposition is profiled onstage. The conceptualizer makes the speculation based on the evidence "Firesorb™ (火 鹖) 较薄的支架壁(the thinner wall of Firesorb™)" which is highlighted onstage in Example 48. We can see that Chinese discourse producers objectively speculate the possibility of products' excellent performance based on their confidence in the products' unique features.

---

① https://www.microport.com.cn/news/925.html. CFDA is now called National Medical Products Administration (NMPA).

6.5 Contrastive Differences of Grounding Grammar in Promotional Discourses of Medical Devices

Cognitive linguists uphold that meaning is conceptualization. Meaning develops as a result of the construal process from an intentional perspective. Having examined the mental representations of modal verbs' conceptual construal process, we can see how the conceptualizer construes the source and target of the modal force. This part deals with a comparison in terms of modality types and construal elements of modal verbs in English and Chinese MDPNs.

Figure 6-10 shows modality distribution across English and Chinese MDPNs. On the whole, it can be seen that both English and Chinese discourses prefer epistemic and dynamic modality with little involvement of deontic modality, which means that promotional discourse producers regardless of their culture and language mainly express modality by incorporating their own attitudes into known or existing knowledge instead of social regulations. This is reasonable as the use of deontic modality is declining in order to achieve politeness. Epistemic modality is overly used 96 times in English MDPNs while dynamic modality is overly used 84 times in Chinese MDPNs, demonstrating their different tendencies in expressing their attitudes. English discourse producers have more confidence in expressing certainty, whereas Chinese discourse producers believe in their own capability.

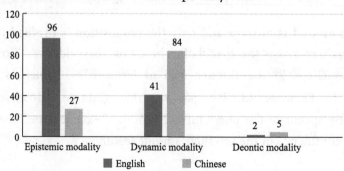

Figure 6-10   Comparison of modality types' distribution

The above analysis revealed that the interpretation of epistemic and dynamic modals from Chinese and English perspectives is rather different in terms of the nature of their conceptual elements as summarized in Table 6-5.

Table 6-5   Summary and comparison of elements in MS and IS scope

Modal verbs	MS	IS
Epistemic "will"	Conceptualizer: we	● Evidence: data, study results; common sense ● Proposition: common practice; study procedure
Dynamic "can"	—	● Trajector: stent, we(conceptualizer) ● Potential acts: excellent performance; contributions
	—	● Trajector: emergent circumstances ● Potential acts: threatening events
Epistemic "may"	—	● Evidence: data, clinical evidence ● Proposition: new practices
Epistemic "could"	—	● Evidence: trial ● Proposition: better performance
Dynamic "能(够) (can)"	—	● Trajector: stent' feature; we(conceptualizer); using stent (condition) ● Potential acts: breakthroughs; excellent performance
Dynamic "可(以) (can)"	—	● Trajector: original products; independent R&D ● Potential acts: breakthroughs
Epistemic "会(will)"	Conceptualizer: we Evidence: expert's explanation; common practice	● Proposition: products' excellent performance
Epistemic "可能(may)"	—	● Evidence: products' features ● Proposition: products' excellent performance

For epistemic modals, both the evidence and the propositions ones are onstage, and they can be objectively construed by readers and become the focus of their attention in the first place. The conceptualizer uses epistemic "will" to make a prediction based on evidence like data or other study results. However, the conceptualizer is in the maximal scope (MS), representing his subjective prediction. Common knowledge like procedures followed by national reimbursement is objectively construed, which equals to a fact. In the meantime, epistemic "may" and "could" are used to objectively make speculation based on evidence from data, clinical evidence, and trials. So epistemic "will" is more subjectively used than epistemic "may" and "could". By contrast, far fewer epistemic modals are employed in Chinese discourses. Epistemic "会 (will)" is employed by discourse producers to predict products' excellent performance based on expert explanation and common practice. And also "可能 (may)" is employed by the discourse producers to boast products' good performance based on the characteristics of the products themselves. Therefore, English discourse producers are data and trial-driven in assessing the likelihood of the potential acts, while Chinese discourse producers are guided by products' features and experts' authorities.

For dynamic modals' conceptual construal, the force implementation process is the focus of attention onstage. Trajector is typically linked to the clausal subject in discourses. In English discourses, the trajector of the force imposed by dynamic "can1" is prototypically associated with products' features, and companies' capabilities. These features are so excellent that they can inevitably produce satisfying treatment effects. However, while exaggerating the companies' capability to ensure continuous quality to serve the patients, the discourse producers show their subjectivity. Dynamic "can2" is used to present possible threatening events and the discourse producers warn it objectively. By contrast, "能(够) (can)" and "可(以) (can)" in Chinese discourses are quite frequently used to impose force coming from products' features, and China's original strengths in R&D. Additionally, potential acts denoted by "可(以) (can)" are objectively construed in order to depict a capable image. There is no doubt that Chinese discourse producers incline to highlight and promote their innovative or original strengths. The development of Chinese medical device companies in the medical fields is still at the infant stage and high-end technological products rely heavily on imports. They are eager to make the world know that they can create their own brands, which will help break the old impression of Chinese products imitating and relying on low prices and low quality to win the market.

As expected, the modal grounding analysis decodes how discourse producers construct discourses in order to leave a trustworthy impression that caters to readers' rooted values and beliefs. Readers' perceptions of the coronary stents can be manipulated as they are more likely to interpret discourses in a way that has been deliberately constructed by discourse producers. Considering the promotional purpose of the discourses and embodied experience of cognitive linguistics, the author discusses the contrastive differences and the possible reasons for similarities and differences revealed in discourses. The overall cognitive mechanisms of English and Chinese medical device promotional discourses are displayed in Figure 6-11 and Figure 6-12.

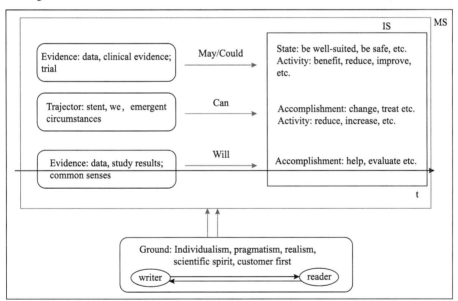

Figure 6-11   Cognitive mechanism in English medical device promotional discourses

As for English MDPNs, for epistemic modal verbs "will", "could", "may", discourse producers make assessments relying on clinical data and common knowledge, depicting well-studied, authorized stents. The reason why the texts are constructed in this way may be that American people foster scientific spirit from Dewey's pragmatism and logical empiricism. Discourse producers embed such views into their texts to let readers easily trust what is being promoted because they share the same norms and expectations. Discourse producers also manage to get readers more convinced of the magic performance depicted by the accomplishment, activity, and state verbs. These verbs designate changing mental representation of products performance, inducing potential buyers. For dynamic modal verb "can1", the modal force comes from products' features and companies' capabilities which help patients free of untreatable heart diseases. The accomplishment verbs are typically matched to denote good news. "Can2" represents possibilities of emergent circumstances which are the main drivers of purchasing volition, for the activity verbs make people think of the coming of destructive disasters. However, all the salient information represents the conceived reality and unreality in discourse producers' minds.

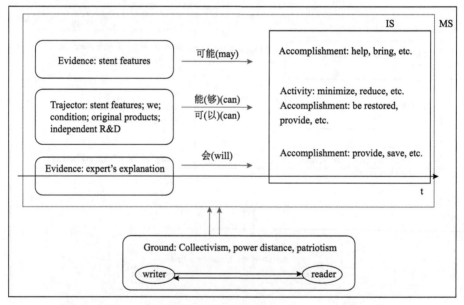

Figure 6-12   Cognitive mechanism in Chinese medical device promotional discourses

As for Chinese MDPNs, for epistemic modal "会 (will)" and "可能(may)", evidence is restricted to the description of products features which are what writers rely on to distinguish themselves from others as they have constantly appeared, and an expert's explanation can prove effectiveness in inducing

Chinese customers as they foster respect for experts' authoritative knowledge. The notable less employment of epistemic modals is attributable to China's collectivistic culture with little tolerance for possible counterarguments. For dynamic modal verbs "能(够) (can)", and "可(以) (can)", products features, technological innovation ability are highlighted, constructing capable stents and innovative companies. It attracts buyers not only by promoting the advantages of products but also by inspiring patriotism. Serving as reference points, the modals situate profiled process designated by these verbs in unreality, persuading potential customers in a more acceptable way.

6.6 Summary

The above analyses have important implications for how domestic medical device companies approach the international market by designing promotional news releases to acquire and retain customers or other concerned parties. Firstly, discourse producers have to be fully aware of foreigners' way of thinking, cultural inheritance, values, beliefs and so on, which contribute to the interpretation of the information presented. Secondly, fancy language is not only restricted to evaluative resources, but also accomplishment and activity verbs which are effective in describing a good product. In order to avoid discomfort caused by blatant or straight promotion, modal verbs and their forms should be selectively used to counterbalance the over-promotion expressed by fancy and exaggerating expressions. Modal verbs are used to weaken absoluteness, demonstrate objectiveness, and show politeness. Thirdly, modal verbs as grounding elements are useful in giving readers the right to participate in the interpretation of discourses to solicit acceptance. In a word, Chapter VI helps to solve real-world problems faced by discourse producers with the mechanisms for them to well organize the content and select linguistic structures in writing promotional texts. Chinese discourse producers have to bear in mind that to be persuasive, they have to show what they have done in doing clinical research, gaining international recognition, putting customers first, and achieving objectivity and capability.

Chapter 7

Cross-cultural Comparison of Cognitive Grammar in Medical Promotional Discourses

The world we see is not predetermined, but is subject to the perspective of the conceptualizers themselves, the way of construal. By concerning with risks and challenges we face when constructing repositories of cognitive expressions in discourses, we need to provoke how insights gained in the course of contrastive research can facilitate the work on such a repository, i.e. how it can, if not completely eliminate, then at least alleviate certain risks and challenges. Therefore, the processes profiled within the attentional scope are essential to the understanding of discourse producers' intentions. This research adopts a CG approach to medical promotion texts by analysing the word grammar in discourses cross-culturally. Through penetrating the medical industries and their official promoting discourses, the author ends up with an in-depth discussion on the cognitive mechanism embedded in Chinese and English medical promotional discourses respectively.

7.1   Cross-linguistic Variations in Cognitive Grammar

When readers read promotional discourses, they are in some sense trying to understand them. But to understand a text completely would be to arrive at its true meaning, and since meaning is always particular and situational (in other words, what a discourse means depends on who has written it, why, when, who is reading, and so on), this is essential. Analyses of discourses are always partial and provisional. Any particular motivation in a discourse presupposes a communicative world, a pattern of cognition and a projection of sociolinguistics.

With regard to cross-linguistic variations in cognitive grammar, the research tackles the cognitive and discoursal differences which depend on the cognitive grammar primarily (but not exclusively) embedded in writers' minds. Consequently, the analytical sections document various discourses related to medical products and services which are recurrent in the promotion business. The research is sensitive to the linguistic requirements of the commodity marketers who want to know the practical benefits that emerge from this kind of discourse study on promotions.

To communicate with the world, text writers manipulate verbal expressions through forms of nouns and verbs to organize their intentions and motivations as well, setting up descriptive frameworks alternative to the mainstream generative cognitive models in various cultures, and offering a unified account of cognitive structure, processing and discourses. By focusing on cognitive grammar, the study illustrates a selection of cognitive abilities and models relevant to grammatical issues, the characterization of word classes and grammatical functions, and the issue of the relation between constituency and dynamicity. To be more specific, text writers apply patterns of neural activation, and conceptualize the word grammar as a cognitive inventory of conventional linguistic units or devices in discourses. The selection of a linguistic unit or device, associated with a specific grammatical pattern, is a pattern of neural activation that can occur more or less unconsciously or automatically, which is entrenched and considered as a cognitive pattern in cultures. Various cognitive patterns are shared by a community of speakers and writers in specific cultures, and constitute images or inventories which hearers and readers can draw from for elaboration and extension which further constitute their new images and inventories.

Essentially, discourses that have linguistic units that have grammatical status are not limited to what is traditionally known as language grammar but may include larger expressions. For instance, the EFFECT FOR CAUSE metonymy "疗效显著 has prominent curative effects" in Chinese discourse provides confidence in the medicine to the patient as the elaboration and extension of readers who frame their positive cognition on the cancer medicine produced by pharmaceutical factories. Whether curative effects are real or not depends on producing entities or institutions instead of the objective doctors or patients who actually use the medicine. While in English discourses, a causational clause also implies an image and further promotes its Anti-Cancer medicine by using "a majority of individuals face a poor prognosis", which elaborates that the dearth of treatment methods for cancer is a serious problem, emphasizing the necessity and significance of the new medicine as an extension. The subject "a majority of individuals" indicates individual patients as the subjects who are the direct users of the medicines. Although the linguistic units, such as the use of metonymic expression of EFFECT FOR CAUSE, are projected with different subjects and their functions embedded. Influenced by linguistic and cultural differences, the Chinese and American writers utilize metonymic subjectivity in Anti-Cancer medicine promotional discourses, possessing an entirely different set of values, norms and social customs in their discourses. Chinese promotional discourse writers to some extent tend to believe in authority and value the reputation and fame of medicine producers a lot, whilst English promotional discourses writers to some extent tend to believe in concrete facts by applying medicine users as examples in discourses, which generates tendencies to select different metonymy types and points of view in Anti-Cancer medicine promotional discourses.

Analysis of stimuli in force dynamics shows that both Chinese and English writers are more likely to use positive stimuli to achieve their promotion. The entities that emit positive stimuli, namely the Antagonist in force-dynamic model, tend to present good and positive aspects, for instance, a new service launched by the company, or the achievements and values of the company. According to the moves identified by move structure analysis, it can be seen that Chinese and English discourse producers usually employ linguistic stimuli containing "force" in Move 2 "establishing backgrounds", Move 3 "introducing the offer", and Move 4 "establishing credentials" rather than other moves. Although the force positions are slightly different, both Chinese and English discourse producers hope to use positive or negative stimuli in these three important moves to highlight the advantages of their medical services and convey goodwill to readers. Furthermore, the constructing processes of cognitive frame consisting of discoursal and word grammar dimensions present that whether it is the communicative purposes the discourse producers want to convey or it is the linguistic stimuli they want to use, they are intended to form fixed frames in the minds of readers, so that the readers can comprehend the services offered by a company in a positive light. Readers decode and process the information they receive from the promotional discourses in the "black box" in the cognitive frame. Through the analyses of stimuli in move structures, different but positive cognition can be formed in Chinese and English readers.

Through modal grounding analysis, the quantitative result shows that the English and Chinese discourse producers prefer epistemic and dynamic modalities with little involvement in deontic modality. Particularly, epistemic modality is overly used in English discourses while dynamic modality is overly used in Chinese discourses. English modal verb "will" accounts for about 35.97%, showing great certainty and confidence. Chinese modal verb "能(够) (can)" accounts for about 43.10%, demonstrating capability. Qualitative analysis of epistemic modal verbs indicates that English discourse producers are data and trial driven and tend to refer to common knowledge in assessing the likelihood of propositions by supporting with facts and statistics, while Chinese discourse producers are product feature-oriented and expert authority-oriented by using a describing way mostly. No scientific result is disclosed at the most salient place. Qualitative analysis of dynamic modal verbs explicates that the profiled roles of the source, target and agent are unified as the trajector which is typically linked to the clausal subject in discourses. The modal force of dynamic "can1" in English discourses is prototypically associated with products' innate excellent features and companies' capabilities. Dynamic "can2" is used to present possible threatening events which can be prevented by using stents. However, in Chinese discourses, "能(够) (can)" and "可(以) (can)" are quite frequently used to impose force coming from product excellent features, and original strength in R&D.

The diversity of languages is not a diversity of signs, sounds and calligraphies, but a diversity of values, thinking patterns and cultural norms. To further elaborate this view in cognitive field, the author argues that the diversity of language is not a diversity of use of lexis and grammars but a diversity of cognition embedded within the lexis and grammars. In the Sapir-Whorf theory, language both expresses cultural patterns and worldviews, and influences habitual ways of thinking in individual members of the speech community. Such "predisposition", it should be noted, does not imply a limitation of thought by language. However, Gumperz and Levinson (1996: 2) claim that the notion of a dynamic, triadic relationship in which "language, thought, and culture are deeply interlocked" is reduced and simplified to a dyadic and unidirectional linguistic determinism and the determination of individual thought expressed by language (Sinha 2021). The reference to culture, which refers to language and "world views", is downplayed in the specific problem fields regarding individual cognitive functions (Sinha & Jensen de Lóprz 2000). This reduction not only distorts the representations of applied linguistics in reality, but also exaggerates cultural differences in language use. The grammar used in discourses, such as modal verbs in both Chinese and English discourses, is not markedly different in texts for promotion purposes, instead, different types and positions of modal verbs, and their evaluation and interpretations are not equivalent in Chinese and English texts and arrive at somewhat different cognition of the promoted products.

This study shows how grammar affects meaning construction in different ways in both English and Chinese. Although some types of cross-linguistic variations in cognitive grammar are fairly unlikely to lead to misinterpreting and misunderstanding, the author has explored, within medical promotional discourses, variations in the ways in which grammar is used in pragmatic inferencing and promoting acts, and variations in the ways in which cognitive grammars relate to business intentions and motives across cultures and languages. The differences are unlikely to present serious problems in cross-linguistic communication through translation. However, the readers' consuming behaviour might be affected when their cognitive processes fail to provide sufficient information for constructing their understanding of the products or services. Thus, cognitive linguistic studies, including semantics and grammars, can be attributed to the economy with which meanings and concepts can be expressed with specific commercial intentions and motives.

7.2 Reasons behind the Misunderstanding of Cognitive Grammar in Cross-linguistic and Cross-cultural Communication

Language delivers ideas, opinions, or ideologies; discourses, as the carrier of language, are embodied with human cognition, demonstrating attitudes, beliefs and values toward the world. Understanding the meaning of the discourse, therefore, involves more than decoding the surfaced structure and literal meaning; it also involves the identification of the "embodied mind" beneath the discourse. Generally, cognitive grammar takes issues with the traditional building-block view of meaning construction, namely the claim that meaning is by and large compositional. Instead, as Broccias (2021) claims, cognitive grammar claims that words are merely prompts for activating a rich array of knowledge domains, parts of which can be combined quite flexibly and creatively. In cross-cultural circumstances, word classes (e.g. metonymies, modal verbs) and grammatical functions (e.g. subjects and verb phrases) are not primitive notions but definable.

The present study presents a scenario for the study of cognitive grammar in medical promotion which provides a commercial context for the readers to infer the intended message. However, in some discourse exempts, the intended meaning may not be immediately obvious as there are insufficient grammar clues to allow the reader to disambiguate the possible cognitive senses for understanding and interpreting the discourses. The analyses of this book reveal that the WG is applied in both Chinese and English, which can be attributed to commercial, communicative, cultural and social features of Eastern and Western cultures.

7.2.1 Commercial and communicative factors

As Kaur et al. (2013: 64) put forward that language in promotion is used to control people's minds as they believe that "the types of verbs used, tenses, active or passive sentences, parallelism, pronouns, modality, nominalizations have an important function in representing 'reality'". In other words, it is not a matter of what is true but a matter of what it is perceived to be true through different language forms.

The first shared major aspect across the two discourses lies in the modal verb forms. The verbs, followed by modals, are mainly accomplishment and activity verbs. As many researchers have studied, discourse producers positively exaggerate products' unique features and excellent performance for the sake of promotion through evaluative languages such as adjectives, quantifier terms etc. (Izquierdo & Blanco 2020). As a supplement, accomplishment and activity verbs represent dynamic ongoing processes, through which readers can be led to imagine a perfect image of a product. Improvements in terms of product performance, treatment, scientific results, etc., are considered to be the primary driver of purchasing behaviour. It can be explained through the communication goals that MDPNs should not only be scientific and credible, but also persuasive and attractive for the purpose of growing sales. The exaggeration of benefits enhances the image that these products can offer a solution to enduring heart diseases. For example, the use of NeoVas stent can be replaced for free for the rest of the years. In addition, both dynamic modals' force across the two corpus comes from and highlights products' features as self-promotion helps to attract consumers in order to show them how they can benefit from the products and the brands.

Communication needs should be a concern. Linguistic strategies such as modalities should be used to counterbalance over-promotion to appeal to caution as modal verbs are the most used uncertainty makers. They are even considered as a tool to show politeness to maintain a good interpersonal relationship (Vergaro 2004). Such an intention can be confirmed as there is no deontic modality appeared. The lower epistemic value denotes more politeness and thus readers have more free choices (Zhao & Feng 2012). Modal verbs are highly grammatical verbs with prominent cognitive features in language as demonstrated in the above analysis. Their semantic function is manifested in grounding analysis, which expresses discourse producers' cognitive control of meanings and public ideologies. It means that the world is just a portion of the mental universe that we conjure up. English and Chinese discourse producers are employing modal verbs' semantic function of reality perception to minimize absoluteness and avoid further responsibility in order to protect themselves.

7.2.2 Cultural and social factors

For cognitive linguistics, language is embodied as it is grounded in our physical, bodily experiences as human beings. Some social and cultural influences have a dominant power in shaping the linguistic system. People constantly see how discourse communities sometimes attach a particular cognitive meaning to a given word or phrase and how it can, at times, be misunderstood or interpreted in different ways by readers outside that discourse community. The present study of this book focuses on the word grammar that is employed by writers in promotional discourses of different cultures with similar attention or motivation for their product or service, and the interpreting problems of promotional discourses can arise when these two cultures come into contact with one another. The problems become even more acute when people from different linguistic or cultural backgrounds need to communicate with another one because regional and national cultures develop particular cognitive patterns that help define their cultural and even discoursal identities.

In this book, the author discusses the word grammar in cross-cultural and cross-linguistic communication, and outlines how word grammar, such as modal verbs in grounding contexts, impedes or facilitates interpreting and understanding between people who have different cultural and linguistic backgrounds. For instance, in Chapter 6, the first sharp difference revealed in English and Chinese medical promotional MDPNs is the top distribution of modality type with 96 (69.06%) occurrences of English epistemic modality and 84 occurrences (72.41%) of Chinese dynamic modality. This can be explained from a cultural perspective. "The cultural environment, either physical or social, leads to differences in perceptual processes" (Nisbett & Miyamoto 2005: 472). Differences between Chinese and English promotional discourses are to some extent due to the orientations of collectivism and individualism. To many Americans, the questioning of one's own and others' ideas or beliefs and engaging in argumentation and debate are regarded as common practice for knowledge construction (Peng & Nisbett 1999: 747). English discourse producers may believe that the use of epistemic modals is necessary to reflect the tentativeness of their claims and to leave them open for discussion. Hyland (1998) argues that hedge words such as modal "may" indicate a weakening of a claim and that the statements presented are opinions rather than accredited facts. That is why epistemic modality is overly used in English discourses. However, most Chinese favour modesty and harmony rather than disputation. Peng and Nisbett (1999) also claim that Chinese culture is to some extent characterized by the belief that debate and argumentation could be meaningless for understanding truth and reality. Some Chinese discourse producers hesitate to use epistemic modals.

Modals' conceptualization reveals the expressions reflected by the source and target of modal forces. The force implementation process is onstage within the focal prominence. What we primarily want to talk about is the focused elements such as "profile and trajectory" (Langacker 2008: 333). The analyses of modals illustrate that English discourse producers are mainly data and trial driven, while Chinese discourse producers are driven by products' intrinsic features and expert authority. This cognitive salience is also culturally based. A scientific way of thinking can find its trace in Dewey's pragmatism and logical empiricism (Richardson 2002). Promoting clinical investigations is the major characteristic of English MDPNs. All the sophisticated devices rely on rigorous application of scientific methods and clear-headed logic. For the Chinese side, power distance involves the extent to which the less powerful members of organizations and institutions accept and view as inequality in power, wealth, and prestige. In purchasing professional devices, Chinese buyers tend to believe in the authority of experts in a specific field, who to some extent represent erudites.

Some social concerns can be accounted for the cognitive rationale. The trajector is typically represented by stents' excellent features and companies' capabilities in both Chinese and English discourses. They play a fundamental role in attracting potential customers and buyers. Sometimes English discourses emphasize emergent circumstances by exaggerating threatening moments. Instead of introducing products' features, another important aspect is to directly point out life-threatening situations to build a badly frightening atmosphere, which is one of the very effective tools to persuade patients to find solutions eagerly. Upholding "customer first", discourses hold customers' attention tightly by leading them to position themselves in such a condition. By contrast, the image of "created in China" repeatedly appears in the locus of attention profiled by modal verbs. Since the image of "made in China" has been rooted in foreigners' minds, there is no wonder that the Chinese side strives to constantly challenge themselves to make breakthroughs. It invokes patriotism in every Chinese citizen who embraces those companies contributing to the nation. The promotion of China's original R&D and Chinese original products is indispensable for "China-created" products to win the international market.

7.2.3   Cognitive factors

The research results in this book provide critical cognitive linguistic analyses for cross-cultural media discourse studies from the perspective of cognitive grammar, based on the theories and methods from applied linguistics, humanities and social and cognitive sciences. Social cognition is constructed through multidisciplinary collaboration. The repository in the empirical studies of cross-linguistic comparison of cognitive grammar can certainly be beneficial because it provides the necessary systematicity, i.e. after understanding the word grammar application within a repository and the way it relates to other words in sentences, communicators can better calibrate their comprehension of the word grammar's counterpart in another language and consequently they can better understand cross-linguistic equivalences. While point of view, force dynamic and modal verbs work on metonymies, frames and groundings, the word grammar has an operational nature that predicate-argument relations and topological arrangement do not have. The latter are ways of organizing knowledge arising from our communication with the world; the former, by contrast, is a matter of re-construal or re-interpretation of organized knowledge by integrating communicators' cognitive construction in different ways. In the case of metonymy, the source provides a point of view of access to the target domain, as a result of the cognitive process, the target is seen from the perspective of the source. From the analyses and discussion on the word grammar applied in medical promotional discourses, it follows that metonymy, word selections and modal verbs cannot be ranked on a par with points of view, frames and grounding since the former three are constructed on the basis of the latter three and the former three involve re-construing pre-existing cognitive ideas rather than just organizing ideas. In other words, word grammar and its applications and interpretations are cognitive operations whose activity ranges over cognitive processes. The book, thus, proves that it is possible to identify different kinds of cognitive process and cognitive model types on which they can operate by looking into interpretive uses of language across cultures.

We can never be sure that a repository of cognitive expressions in a specific culture can be identified in another culture for a number of reasons. This may simply stem from the fact that a language is always in a constant state of flux, innovating itself, which also applies to the system of cognitive expressions which may be continually enriched by not only adding new expressions, or shedding some, but also due to the cross-cultural communication in Internet era in which people are exposed to more cross-cultural differences easily and widely. The cognitive grammar models identified in the present studies of the book prove the cognitive gap cross-culturally, which embeds linguistic construal and description within its communicative framework. The descriptive and explanatory apparatus of the cognitive models is sensitive to promotional discourses and pragmatic categories like cognitive frame and illocutionary meanings of force dynamics and modal verbs.

Cognitive competence and operations are essential for filling the cognitive gap as a part of mental equipment. They are mechanisms that our minds use in order to communicate our intentions and motives beyond the language we use, and also make mental representations. Cognitive competence concerns knowledge obtained directly and indirectly, memory storage and retrieval, cognition and recognition, experienced and learned, and the like, and how their operations have a direct relationship with the mind's ability to construe, represent, and reason about the world. In language-based communicative contexts, cognitive grammar together with cognitive semantics are essential to forming the parts of the mental mechanisms that allow discourse users to variously access, select, quote, and integrate conceptual and cognitive structure as needed for discoursal production and interpretation purposes. The cognitive models license processes of cognitive activities on the basis of linguistic preferences and habituation. Such typical examples can be identified in the analyses and discussion of the word grammar used by Chinese and English discourse writers to construct different cognitive processes and patterns. Given the general nature of linguistic differences, the author devotes her effort to generating five cognitive activities in which the cognitive competencies need.

1. Quote

Quoting is regarded as the most directly and subconsciously cognitive activity of the five. Such an activity provides a basic concept that the discourse writers can acquire from other sources, such as institutions, professionals and academic studies.

Example 49 (Source: ET24)

... in patients who received <u>VENCLYXTO plus rituximab, resulting in</u> <u>an 83 percent reduction in the risk of disease progression or death</u> (hazard ratio [HR]: 0.17; 95% confidence interval [CI]: 0.11-0.25; $P<0.0001$). (AbbVie Receives European Commission Approval of VENCLYXTO® (venetoclax) Plus Rituximab for the Treatment of Patients with Chronic Lymphocytic Leukemia Who Have Received at Least One Prior Therapy, PR Newswire, 1 November, 2018)[①]

Example 50 (Source: CT8)

中山大学肿瘤防治中心张力教授团队研究证实,<u>国产 PD-1 免疫治疗</u><u>药物卡瑞利珠单抗对复发转移的鼻咽癌疗效显著。</u>(鼻咽癌治疗获新突破 国产 PD-1 治疗鼻咽癌将给患者带来福音,**恒瑞医药/新华网**,2018 年 9 月 29 日)[②]

The research conducted by Professor Zhang's team from Sun Yat-Sen University Cancer Centre (SYSUCC) has confirmed that domestic PD-1 immunotherapy medicine Camrelizumab has prominent curative effect on the recurrence and metastasis of nasopharyngeal cancer. (New breakthrough in

① https://www.prnewswire.com/news-releases/abbvie-receives-european-commission-approval-of-venclyxto-venetoclax-plus-rituximab-for-the-treatment-of-patients-with-chronic-lymphocytic-leukemia-who-have-received-at-least-one-prior-therapy-300741883.html

② http://m.xinhuanet.com/health/2018-09/29/c_1123504909.htm

nasopharyngeal cancer treatment: domestic PD-1 treatment of nasopharyngeal cancer brings good news to patients, Hengrui Pharma/Xinhua Net, 29 September, 2018)

The English discourse producer uses $X_4Y_2Z_4$ and $X_4Y_2Z_3$ **viewpoints** in Example 49 to quote the intended result which shows that the patients who receive VENCLYXTO plus rituximab are actually 83 percent less likely to have a cancer progression or death, which was provided by the pharmaceutical company AbbVie. This direct quotation explicitly indicates that the positive effects and outcomes are brought to the patients by the new drug combination, while in Example 50, the Chinese discourse writer uses $X_2Y_4Z_4$ and $X_2Y_4Z_3$ **viewpoints** to quote "国产 PD-1 免疫治疗药物卡瑞利珠单抗对复发转移的鼻咽癌疗效显著…domestic PD-1 immunotherapy medicine Camrelizumab has prominent curative effect on the recurrence and metastasis of nasopharyngeal cancer", applying CAUSE and EFFECT metonymy to build patients' confidence on the medicine.

The direct application of quotation, based on the information supplied by pharmaceutical companies, composes the core of CAUSE and EFFECT metonymies "reduction" and "curative effect", constructing the intended persuasive activity regardless of the linguistic differences in PoV applications. Direct quotations used by discourse writers are often related to professional knowledge beyond their cognition, which is necessary to construct metonymies that indicate persuasive information about the treatment results.

2. Access

Accessing indicates the information that can be easily reached, understood and used and so on. Such a cognitive activity consists in applying access to the most relevant concepts and ideas on the basis of textual information which discourse readers often have no difficulties in comprehending because of shared common knowledge.

Example 51 (Source: ET3)

COVID-19 is at the fore-front but major <u>healthcare problems</u> [Ago] related to chronic disease, lack of access to care and other health care challenges, can be more effectively **addressed with** <u>continuous care</u> [Ant]. (SteadyMD Telemedicine Doctors Provide Alternative to Face-to-Face Clinical Visits for COVID-19 Concerns, SteadyMD, 11 March, 2020)[①]

Example 52 (Source: CT6)

<u>规范化诊疗以及长期个体化的健康管理方案</u>[Ant]，可以做到精准筛查，也可以大大**阻止**<u>病情</u>[Ago]进一步恶化，提高慢阻肺患者生活质量。（平安好医生与勃林格殷格翰深度合作，打造中国首个线上慢阻肺全方位管理项目，平安好医生/勃林格殷格翰，2020 年 7 月 9 日）[②]

<u>Standardized treatment and long-term individualized health management programs</u> [Ant] can achieve accurate screening and greatly **prevent** <u>further deterioration of the sickness</u> [Ago], improving the life quality of COPD patients. (PING AN Good Doctor and Boehringer Ingelheim have cooperated deeply to create China's first online COPD comprehensive management project, PING AN Good Doctor / Boehringer Ingelheim, 9 July, 2020)

In force dynamic grammatical context, the Ago expression "healthcare problems" in Example 51 can be easily accessed from various news reports worldwide, while the Ago expression "further deterioration of the sickness" in Example 52 is a common sense which directly related to poor health management. It is easy for discourse readers to find the interrelationship between the Ago and Ant. In the two examples, both Chinese and English discourse writers apply the stronger force with "Antagonist+" pattern to address health management programs and the coronal pandemic which can effectively stimulate readers' cognition on the sickness.

The process of accessing, on account of the common knowledge supplied by the public, such as schools, institutions or propaganda, is transparent and open to everyone who can easily acquire the information, needs rational efforts. Such a cognitive activity is often universal, collective and common for both discourse writers and readers, which often provides a basis for the latter cognitive activities, such as selection, substitution and integration.

---

① https://www.steadymd.com/2020/03/11/steadymd-telemedicine-doctors-provide-alternative-to-face-to-face-clinical-visits-for-covid-19-concerns/

② https://www.boehringer-ingelheim.cn/press-releases/ping-an-hao-yi-sheng-yu-bo-lin-ge-yin-ge-han-shen-du-he-zuo-da-zao-zhong-guo-shou-ge-xian-shang-man-zu-fei-quan-fang-wei-guan-li-xiang-mu

3. Select

Selecting is regarded as the first personally and consciously cognitive activity related to access through which its process allows discourse writers to pick out relevant linguistic devices and information from the conceptual package they have obtained from their learning and studies, and allows the discourse readers to interpret discourses based on their mental work and degrees of digestion and assimilation. Such an activity is activated and aided by linguistic expressions and interpretations which are linked with contexts and personal learning experience of discourse writers/readers.

Example 53 (Source: ET19)

The XIENCE stent is used in life-saving treatments that **can** help prevent or treat heart attacks and has now consistently been proven safe with short DAPT strategies for HBR patients. (Abbott's XIENCE™ Stent Receives European Approval for One-Month Dual Anti-Platelet Therapy (DAPT) for High Bleeding Risk Patients, Abbott Laboratories, April 6, 2021)[①]

Example 54 (Source: CT2)

Firesorb™（火鹮）较薄的支架壁厚度使产品的通过外径得以减少，并**可能**缩短降解时间，有效降低血栓形成的风险。(业内第二代生物全可吸收血管支架系统 Firesorb™（火鹮）通过 CFDA 创新医疗器械特别审批申请，微创，2016 年 6 月 13 日)[②]

The thinner wall of Firesorb™ reduces the crossing profile of the product, and **may** shorten the degradation time, effectively reducing the risk of thrombosis. (The industry's second-generation biological fully absorbable vascular stent system Firesorb™ has passed the special approval application for CFDA innovative medical devices, MicroPort, 13 June, 2016）

Compare Example 53 and Example 54, modal selection demonstrates discourse writers' desires and motives to influence readers' interpretations of the contexts and reality. In Example 53, the subject "XIENCE stent" indicates

---

① https://abbott.mediaroom.com/2021-04-06-Abbotts-XIENCE-TM-Stent-Receives-European-Approval-for-One-Month-Dual-Anti-Platelet-Therapy-DAPT-for-High-Bleeding-Risk-Patients

② https://www.microport.com.cn/news/925.html

that the internal feature of the stent gives itself the modal force and carries out the potential action with permissive meaning, showing higher reliability of the product. If the writer changes "can" to "may", its deontic modality would be interpreted as an epistemic modality with a speculative meaning. Then its reliability degree would not be considered very high by readers. Similarly, in Example 54, "可能 (may)" shows the construal process of epistemic modality, through which the discourse writer wants to speculate the performance of "the thinner wall of Firesorb™" is not 100% safe. But if the discourse writer selects "可以 (can)", he or she intends to implant deontic modality, revealing a much higher safety for the performance and quality of "the thinner wall of Firesorb™" which is mostly unable to keep promise. Such selections will influence readers' comprehension of the product and certainly their consumption behaviour.

Cognitive selection plays an overwhelmingly strong intended role in meaning construction that leads readers to call upon a situation that obeys two requirements: on the one hand, it is conceptually consistent with the in-built meanings provided by the word grammar, such as the in-built degrees and possibilities provided by modals; on the other hand, whether there is any linguistic distraction or alteration which may show different orientations, such as the ambiguity and fuzziness in interpretations of the word grammar. This involves a selection of conceptual structure to satisfy the writers' intention of description because of the sensitive selection of the cognitive construction in the discourses. The default interpretation of the modal meanings, for instance, is that of the complaint by the product users if there is any. To avoid default interpretation, the discourse writers are required carefully to consider the selection of the word grammar that should be consistent with the readers' cognitive actions.

4. Integrate

Integration, also called "blending" proposed by Fauconnier and Turner (1996, 1998, 2002), is a comprehensive and cognitive activity in which conceptual structure is a common cognitive process that underlies much of human creative thinking and reasoning. Cognitive integration consists of the guided combination of selected conceptual structure, which replies to the previous three cognitive activities as described above. The integrating activity involves combination, elaboration, extension and creation.

Example 55 (Source: ET2)

Historically, a majority of these individuals do not receive treatment and face a poor prognosis. (U.S. FDA Approves DAURISMO™ (glasdegib) for Adult Patients with Newly-Diagnosed Acute Myeloid Leukemia (AML) for Whom Intensive Chemotherapy is Not an Option, Pfizer, 21 November, 2018)[1]

The expression of "a majority of... individuals... and face a poor prognosis" in Example 55 presents an integrating process which can be sketched in Figure 7-1.

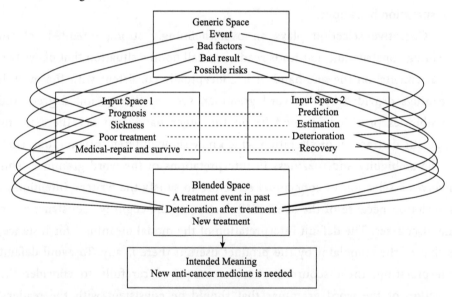

Figure 7-1　Conceptual integration network of "face a poor prognosis"

The integrating process suggests that the lack of treatment methods is a serious problem, emphasizing the great necessity and significance of the new medicine DAURISMO. Similarly, the discourse readers may find it easier to

① https://www.pfizer.com/news/press-release/press-release-detail/u_s_fda_approves_daurismo_glasdegib_for_adult_patients_with_newly_diagnosed_acute_myeloid_leukemia_aml_for_whom_intensive_chemotherapy_is_not_an_option

accept this opinion since they, as individuals of a majority of cancer patients, take the agent's view, which may lead them to expect new medicine and new treatment for a better prognosis (event). Thus, an EVENT FOR SUBEVENT metonymy "face a poor prognosis", which may comprise of several events like facing negative outcomes, losing faith and getting worse, provides the reader with mental assessment to the issue of how bad AML patients can get without proper drug therapy. In combination and elaboration of the semantic implication of metonymy "face a poor prognosis", such a grammatical construction emphasizes the great necessity and significance of the new medicine DAURISMO, and therefore helps the promotion of this new medicine to AML patients.

Conceptual integration can similarly be identified in Chinese promoting discourses but with different interpretations in input spaces 1 and 2, and certainly develops differently in blended space and intended meaning. For instance, $X_2Y_4Z_4$ and $X_2Y_4Z_3$ PoVs, as a bird's eyes angle and a medium or long shot distance showing through The EVENT FOR SUBEVENT metonymy, can present a fusion which the word grammar functions as one of integration by combination and elaboration. It should be noted that for integration, the event described in the integrated process often frequently co-occurs in people's experience, otherwise, the content of input spaces 1 and 2 in the integrating processes would demonstrate dynamically and bring about different blended meanings and intended meanings.

7.3   Cognitive Grammar and Language Evaluation and Position

The theory of word grammar initially receives its name for its rejection of phrase structure (Hudson 1984), but later its focus on language has broadened from syntax to semantics, morphology, sociolinguistics, historical linguistics, language learning and language processing since then. Traditional approaches to grammar have paid more attention to language forms, structures and the description or interpretation of the internal relationship, and traditional contrastive analysis only studies the differences in the form of language, not the reason causing the differences, whereas cognitive contrastive analysis pays more attention to the reasons from the perspective of cognition. However, the approaches to grammar based on cognition lay full emphasis on the functions of the cognitive subjects. Cognitive approaches to grammar focus directly upon the linguistics system. In this book, the author analyses Chinese grammar from integrated perspectives (e.g. discourse study, cognitive linguistics, and lexical study), which combines the essence of Western approaches to grammar for the sake of giving an explanatory study about grammar and its usage in texts and possible impacts on readers' cognitive and ideological construction in reality, not simply the pragmatic studies in academic fields.

In an overview of WG suggested by Joseph and Droste (1991), the most obviously non-standard feature of WG is that it deals with the whole of syntax without referring to anything but words—the notions "phrase", "clause" and even "sentence" plays no part in a WG grammar. According to WG, dependency relations between words are basic and constituents grouped around words are derivative, whereas phrase structure grammar assumes that the relation between constituent structure and dependency is the other way around. Another noteworthy characteristic of WG syntactic structure is that grammatical relations are also taken as basic, rather than as derivative. Moreover, grammatical relations are viewed as organized hierarchically. So in this way, WG integrates two well-established grammatical ideas, namely dependency and grammatical relations. Features are in fact used in WG syntax, but only in the narrowly restricted domain of morpho-syntactic features. In this study, the author proves that, within the WG analytical scope, dependency relations between words are basic, and constituents grouped around words are derivative, whereas phrase structure grammar assumes that the relation between constituent lexis, move and structure and their inter-dependency is evident and requisite. Besides, WG and its grammatical relations are viewed as discourse organization and meaning control. So in this way, WG integrates two well-established grammatical ideas, namely dependency and grammatical relations. Discourse meanings and features are in fact used in WG patterns.

Word grammar, thus, is a model of discoursal analysis based on the following assumptions in this book.

1) Except in coordinate structures, the largest grammatical unit is the

words or word phrases.

2) There is inter-dependence between word selections and their applied typologies, forms and tenses in discourses.

3) WG grammar is a set of propositions defining relationships among entities, actions, events, the most important of these relationships being those of construals of discoursal compositions and instantiation.

4) WG integrates with discourses and determines the construal of conceptualizations of words in discourses.

In brief, WG rejects the traditional and persisting distinction between grammar and lexicon. WG postulates that "Language is a conceptual network" (Hudson 1984) in which each network element—whether a word or a word property—possesses connections of various sorts, both semantic and syntactic, to one or more other elements, such as word formation, word creation, motivation for words or even dialect syntax. As Hudson (2007) sees it, the "new" WG should expand its embrace of experimental psychology which has determined the linguistic and other cognitive processing, especially in its incorporation of the processes of "spreading activation" and "default inheritance" as the prime sources of dynamism and efficiency in language networks. Word grammar should be one of the cognitive foundations of applied linguistic studies owning to its theoretical bases on cognitive science, its major arguments in linguistics, and its up-to-date explanations for various linguistic phenomena related to language use in reality, such as a number of commonly accepted ideas and facts in related disciplines—activation, attention, chunking, default inheritance logic, episodes, frequency effect, long-term memory and working memory, network, parallel distribution processing, priming, prototypes, schema, scripts, selective memory, and the Stroop effect (Hudson 2010).

Although the principles of WG rest on cognitive science, shedding more light on the process of humans' cognition in language. Furthermore, WG provides a new method and tool for exploring the nature of language and its way of syntactic analysis can be applied in grammar studies and teaching practice. In the era of overwhelming information explosion, institutional discourses act as new and efficient ways for various types of consumers to learn about upcoming products and for companies to promote their products.

A successful discourse can bring companies an incredible reputation, instant feedback and good relationship with their users. Besides, it can help companies to boost their sales. Actually, medical device promotion relies much on print and broadcast advertisements, brochures, pamphlets, websites, conferences, seminars etc. (Conko 2011). The news pages of companies' official websites become the most effective knowledge-transfer tool (William-Jones 2006), through which manufactures make themselves more recognizable, sell their values and compete for health care needs. They, on the one hand, present a full account of information about clinical outcomes, authoritative certification, product launches or other business events. Instead of just circulating knowledge, they also carry promotional purposes as many linguists have identified by examining their generic features (Bhatia 2004; Erjavec 2004; Maat 2007). However, promotional materials which may contain misleading information with regard to the use of medical devices or their properties are strictly prohibited under government regulations and social norms. The attractive language is therefore regulated and it is thus important to explore how these texts operate to influence readers' expectations and decisions.

7.4 Cognitive Problems and Marketing Promotional Discourse Improvement

According to the 2013 China Health Statistics Yearbook, the reform of the economic system has driven the reform of the health care system since the reform and opening up in China, while government medical subsidies to public institutions only account for about 14.65% of their revenues. The ratio of national health expenditure to GDP in the world is shown on the WHO website as follows: "Japan is 8.1%, Germany is 10.4%, France is 11.1%, the UK is 9%, Australia is 8.8%, Sweden is 9.1%, the U.S. is 16.1%, and China is 4.3% in 2010." (Yu & Yue 2011). As the data have revealed, the financial support for health care from Chinese government is far below the world average. The lack of financial support from the government for healthcare, coupled with the market-oriented institutional reform of hospitals, has directly led to the tendency for hospitals to become profit-oriented. Hospitals are constantly raising the prices of medicine and medical services to maintain their own survival and development, while at the same time ignoring the needs of the general public for health care. For a domestic stent, the ex-factory price is only 3,000 yuan, but price in the hospital will be 27,000 yuan; for an imported stent, the CIF (cost, insurance and freight) price is only 6,000 yuan, but the price in the hospital will be 38,000 yuan. High drug prices may not only directly result in the current tension between doctors and patients in China, but also greatly affect the Chinese medical products coming to the world.

If cognitive diversity can be analysed and measured by linguistic devices and their applications that take into account the number and the frequencies of different cultural groups, then, what are the effects of these diversities on market outcomes? This present study reveals that, by focusing on linguistic heterogeneity and cognitive semantics and grammar as the main dimensions, communicators from different cultural backgrounds with different cognitive experiences would be faced with the question of what constitutes the relevant linguistic classification (e.g. metaphor or metonymy) and selections (e.g. modal verbs or noun phrases) from the perspective of cognitive linguistics. In trying to determine the relevant groups to construe meanings of the linguistic devices, the author argues that different cognitive linguistic cleavages may matter for different business and market outcomes. Obviously, shared cognition across cultures would promote business and marketization because of correct interpretation of discourses and satisfaction of personal expectations. As Desmet et al. (2016) propose that coarse linguistic divisions and selections can create conflict and lead to a lack of redistribution of products.   Cognition consolidation and linguistic expressions/discourses are sufficient to generate adverse effects on outcomes such as promoting growth that requires coordination and communication between heterogeneous groups from different cultural backgrounds.

Given economic, technological and cultural changes that corporations have to face while doing international business, corporate discourse writers should adjust to the new cultural environment by involving cognitive factors, such as cognition on globalization, advances in scientific technology, the increasing social responsibility of companies and their great impact on people's lives. The accelerated changes in the business environment together with the constant drive to make huge profits have been obtaining a strong market position, winning new customers and retaining old ones as well. This has made them be aware of the importance of the language they use not only to build self-awareness, but also to construct cognition of readers or potential customers from other cultures. Corporate promotional discourses and their analyses have therefore been enriched by an emphasis on naturally occurring and authentic linguistic data. The amount of internal, external and interactive communicative practices in contemporary enterprises turns corporate discourses into various purposeful discourses that exploit synergies among communication techniques, genres, styles and communication goals in the enterprise. Meanwhile, cross-cultural cognitive discourse studies can help to examine how corporations interact through languages not only with their employees and stakeholders, but also with their target markets, existing customers, and the world at large, and how these corporations' overall public images are shaped internally and externally.

From the analytical results revealed in the book, the author proposes that the construction of cognition by corporations through discourses contains two interrelated ways. One is a cognitive process that encompasses a corporate's promotional intentions, marketing goals, corporate identity and so on, which are maintained through series of institutional discourses embedded with its culture and values. Another one is language pragmatics which are seen as discursive expressions of a corporate's concept of itself as expressed in discourses for target readers in other cultures, such as investors, customers, and the general public. The two interrelated ways help a corporate to construct a positive/negative commercial image in the context of another culture in order to gain legitimacy for its commercial promotion actions. Thus, the corporate promotional discourse, a type of Aristotelian epideixis that embraces utilitarian values and business goals, should create a sense of commonality and shared cognition among the members of the society that the commercial discourses are aimed at not only internal but external readers, who subsequently become likely to accept and support the company's actions, such as products promotion, in different cultural contexts. The commercial credibility of the company and the corporate ethos, is built through cross-cultural cognitive awareness and a combination of proper linguistic applications, communication strategies, ideological mechanisms in discourses. Such an integration in discourses is all designed to create a self-enhancement reputation (through the celebration of "established" or "accepted" to construct public cognition) and self-promotion (through image and identity to construct institutional cognition), thus perpetuating the combination of integrated cognition that allows a company to shirk a veritable rendering of accounts to their target readers at different cultures and professional levels, and as well as the world.

7.4.1　The cognitive problems in cross-cultural communication

Cognitive problems are generally related to cognitive gaps in which the differences are often identified. The misunderstanding and its possible consequences may lead to various commercial disputes and misjudgement. Cognitive behaviour and operations underlie the output of language for communication and are intrinsically related to a number of issues of grammar and lexis used in discourses. In this book, the author has applied a number of ways to use cognitive grammar to identify the across-cultural discoursal differences which might lead to different interpretations and meaning construe. One of the most significant examples of negative consequences of possible cross-cultural misunderstanding involving cognitive semantics identified by Yang (2020: 76) concerning "ARMY metaphor".

Example 56
在政府主导下，以中车四方股份公司等 10 家核心企业为主体，联合我国相关领域优势高校、研究机构和国家级创新平台，组成了世界规模最大的中国高速列车技术创新"**联合舰队**"**(combined fleet)**。(中车四方：自主创新打造中国高铁"金名片"。人民网，2016 年 2 月 28 日)①

Under the guidance of the government, China has formed the world's largest "**combined fleet**" of HSR technology innovation, taken CSR SiFang Co., Ltd and 9 other core enterprises as its main body and combined with universities, research institutes and national innovation platforms in related fields. (CSR SiFang: To create the "golden name card" of China's high-speed rail through independent innovation. People.cn, 28 February, 2016)

---

① https://www.crrcgc.cc/sfgf/g7217/s4940/t264573.aspx

The ARMY metaphor "combined fleet" in Example 56 represents the company or a country at war. The concept of the ARMY in the source domain is thus reflecting an organization, a business type or a country in fierce competition, which joins in the "war" and fights for victory. Misunderstanding can also be related to cognitive construction. Another example, raised by Yang (2020: 86) as an English version of a novel metaphorical use, also demonstrates cross-cultural differences regarding "zero" cognitive construction.

Example 57

A smart but busy man, Mr. Musk announced that he wanted to make Hyperloop a sort of **open-source Manhattan Project** for high-speed transportation, since he didn't have the time to pursue it himself. (Can a 700 M.P.H. Train in a Tube Be for Real? *New York Times*, May 19, 2016)

The "open-source Manhattan Project" in Example 57 as a novel metaphor is interpreted as a complicated and huge project in modern English culture for its leading functions and economic position in the world, which implies that a project cannot be fulfilled by one company or one country. Such a novel metaphor makes a departure from deep-rooted semantic domains, especially in Chinese culture, as "Manhattan Project" is rarely compared to "a company". Since no similarity or correspondence can be recognized, the Chinese are confused about how to relate the "Manhattan Project" to "a high-speed railway company" for no or zero cognitive construction. Because of the cognitive gap existing between cultures, it is hard to reach a mutual understanding of the promoted products cross-culturally.

By using conflicting metaphors, such as ARMY metaphor, or even novel metaphors, the antagonistic effects of the target are emphasized especially in aspects such as aggression, competition, and being confrontational. Thus, to promote products to Western countries, like the U.S., such kind of promoting behaviour would be interpreted and understood negatively; while in China, such an ARMY metaphor would be interpreted positively as a promoting act with joint efforts, functions and power. Yang (2020) found that although both the Chinese and American discourse writers employ conflict metaphors, such as WAR metaphor, ARMY metaphor, readers might construct different cognitions to interpret the organizational promoting purposes and business motives.

Most misunderstandings caused by cognitive semantics and grammar are evident, but they can still interfere with successful communication between individuals with different linguistic and/or cultural backgrounds. Misunderstanding in both cognitive semantics and cognitive grammar may cause misunderstanding of the discourses translated from other cultures. For instance, when faced with a novel metaphor, such as "Manhattan Project", a translator can either translate it directly into the target language as "曼哈顿项目" or find a corresponding target language expression (which may or may not involve a metaphor) as "巨无霸 (a novel Chinese metaphor)/超级项目公司 (an interpretation of the super big company)" that is more culturally appropriate. The two translation strategies are defined as "interlingual" and "intersemiotic" by Jakobson (1971a, 1971b). The first strategy involves the replacement of a verbal sign with another verbal sign belonging to the target language. The latter one, on the other hand, refers to, rather than focusing on the words, the overall message that needs to be conveyed. Thus, "the translator, instead of paying attention to the verbal signs, concentrates more on the information that is to be delivered" (Littlemore 2015: 187). The distinction of the translated version between tight "literal" translation and a looser form of translation that focuses on the overall meaning rather than the words themselves is surely associated with his/her cognition of the "Manhattan Project" in American culture and Chinese linguistic culture.

As with all types of language, one would not expect the same or similar equivalent target version to be appropriate for the source target semantic or grammatical units. In other words, one would also not expect the same and similar equivalent expressions to meet the linguistic need of the target language according to the type of cognitive linguistic element (e.g. cognitive semantic and grammatical expressions) involved, its construal meanings interpreted and the genre and register features of the discourse within which it is found. Cognitive semantics that draw on specific cultural references probably need to be translated loosely with the use of target language equivalents (such as metaphors), whereas cognitive grammars draw on less specific cultural references, which probably needs to be translated more directly for the less culturally bound expressions (such as modal verbs). The semantic, grammatical and their illocutionary differences that are found between languages leave the translators with cognitive construction and linguistic choices as to how close to the original discourses they want to sound in other target cultures.

7.4.2 Discourses enhancement and improvement

Cognitively, corporate promotional discourses are rooted in metaphor, metonymy, image schema, and word grammar as the primary aspects that link words, images, sounds and phrases to positive product characteristics and have the distinct rhetorical functions of having immediate impacts on the readers. However, the author specifies that many promotional discourses in one cultural context cannot convey the same associations in another cultural context, and stresses the need to adapt to the local culture, especially in global promotion actions. Meanwhile, the author also argues that while promotional discourses might have a "distorting effect" in the sense that it is a means of promoting or controlling the ideological values of target readers, the most important element of promotional discourses across cultures is that the promoting aspect, which increasingly permeates other aspects of corporate discourse, such as the informational aspect and persuasive action, shall result in a hybrid nature of discourse. Thus, understanding the differences in cross-cultural communication, in cognitive patterns and how to improve cross-cultural cognition is fundamental to enhance cross-cultural communication awareness and competence. In addition, achieving cognitive and pragmatic cross-cultural adaptation also depends on various linguistic applications for cross-cultural product marketization, such as discoursal strategies and lexical seletions in publicity. Based on Yang (2020) and its research in cross-cultural analysis of cognitive semantics and cognitive syntax, the author has summarized the problems of cognitive construction of business discourse that communicators have often experienced in reality (Figure 7-2).

Cultural perception, language cognition, cultural identity and differences of cognitive pragmatics in cross-cultural commercial product promotion consist of a systematic linguistic project. To achieve cross-cultural language adaptation, discourse writers have to rely on the improvement of cognitive ability and discoursal strategy adjustment in cross-cultural communication.

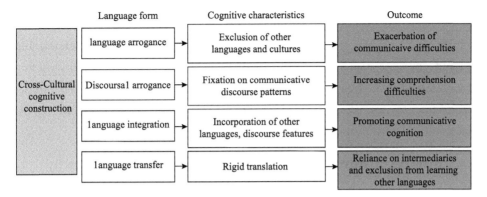

Figure 7-2   Model of cross-cultural cognitive construction

Strategy 1. Identifying linguistic-pragmatic differences and boosting cognitive abilities

When producing discourse, writers are accustomed to predicting the purpose and communicative meaning of other's discourses from their own linguistic habits and discourse positions, and generally based on their own familiar cognitive standards and discourse laws, rather than placing themselves in others discourse situations to deconstruct, reconstruct and interpret the meaning of discourse. Although this behaviour is not unusual in intercultural communication, ignoring the distinctiveness of linguistic cognition of discourse, taking word grammar for an example, will undoubtedly lead to miscognition, misunderstanding, and misinterpretation of a text or an utterance, which in turn will lead to miscommunication. The difficulty of cross-cultural communication lies in the cognitive differences. Therefore, increasing cognitive ability and balancing cognitive differences become the prerequisite for effective communication, while the key to understanding cognitive language in cognitive construction lies in learning to understand their own culture and other culture from a cognitive perspective.

Intercultural communicators, who have a full psychological preparation and cognitive prediction of their own languages and cultures and the possible cognitive competence in the process of intercultural interaction, can construct a reasonable intercultural cognitive model, perceive themselves and their opponents in the discourses, and adjust themselves to the foreign discoursal environment with proper cognitive framing and discoursal strategies. For instance, when promoting Chinese products in other countries, it is not appropriate to perform mere discourse translation or language conversion, but should consider discourse reconstruction problems, cognitive reconstruction problems and language selection problems. This poses relatively higher requirements on discourse, language, and pragmatics to achieve AI intercultural communication.

Strategy 2. Adjusting the discourse strategy to seek empathy

Cross-cultural communicative cognition is the concept formed by a combination of an individual's past insights, experiences, mind thinking, expectations, and evaluations in multicultural communicative contexts. When in the same or similar communicative contexts, the discourse will be produced based on producers' familiar linguistic conventions and previous communicative experiences. When producers lack sufficient linguistic cognition and cultural conceptions of multicultural communicative contexts, the construction of the discourse in their minds will tend to be homogeneous and lack cross-cultural integration, and thus the language choices made will be narrower and more rigid based on their own linguistic experiences. Therefore, by improving the intercultural cognitive level of the discourse producer and understanding the cognitive construction of discourse and language choice in different cultures (e.g. the force dynamics in different moves), the discourse construction and language choice in the mind of the discourse writers will be more diversified, and the discourse will not only be in readers' eyes but also in the hearts, so that the goal of successful communication can be truly achieved, which is the only way to achieve successful communication, and to promote Chinese products globally and be accepted by other countries, and also produce consumer resonance.

Strategy 3. Comprehending cultural cognitive patterns on discourse in other countries and developing consensus

Cognitive ability determines communicative style and language choices. The higher level of cognition is the intensive integration of cognitive commonalities and variabilities. On the basis of understanding cultural and linguistic cognitive differences, it will adjust language usage, discourse structure and cultural adaptation to differences reasonably and effectively. That is, to put oneself in the cognitive position and linguistic perspective of the other party, to use culturally acceptable linguistic strategies, discourse structure and cognitive patterns of the other party, to think what the other party thinks and to develop consensus. The process of writing a discourse is not only about language transfer, but also about thinking "if I were an English speaker, how would I construct the content of the discourse". For example, "I would incorporate different positive lexical items in different steps to achieve promotional purposes"; "If I use metaphors, what spatial point of view should I use"; "When I use modal verbs, how do I achieve the interpersonal effect of communication with native English speakers" and other transpositional approaches.

Strategy 4. Leveraging language advantage to eliminate cultural stereotypes

Chinese products have entered the world market by experiencing the stages of inception, development and prosperity, and more and more Chinese people are also going through the process of being unfamiliar with foreign cultures to cognizing and recognizing them, which is due to the promotion of foreign language teaching, and China's economic reform and her opening up to the outside world. English, as a universal language (Lingua Franca), stands out in its important position in international communication. The overall requirement of English for training talents in our universities and enterprises has enhanced the language basis of our foreign communication and the language ability of cross-cultural communication, thus increasing our communicative confidence. However, in the process of learning and utilizing English, Chinese often rely on traditional cultural thinking and linguistic cognitive patterns. Therefore, due to the existence of a certain gap between our discourse patterns and those of English-speaking countries, despite the daily use of English, the promotion has not only not achieved expected economic benefits, but also even produced a certain amount of misinterpretation and misunderstanding, which forms a more negative stereotype. Consequently, we should have an open and positive mind in cross-cultural communication, understand the language cognitive patterns and discoursal expression habits of different cultures, and interpret different values and ways of thinking from them, so as to achieve the purpose of successful communication and successfully have the world recognize our products again.

In addition, introducing cognitive concepts and cognitive linguistics in foreign or second language teaching can facilitate language learners to use foreign languages more efficiently and accurately, both in discourse and in sentences, grammar, and vocabulary, and to achieve cultural linguistic adaptation at the linguistic level of discourse, utterance, grammar, and lexical items, and to communicate into the mind.

7.5　Summary

In addition to cross-cultural differences in language, cognition and discourse, more social, educational, and individually experiential phenomena should be considered and integrated in one's knowledge for communication across borders and nationalities. Language principles, which result from cultural preferences, and dictate that communication occurring at different levels is more likely to be selected to represent the overall cognitive process than the communication itself occurring in the duration. Many of the language principles are determined by cognitive process and cognitive construction which further determine the language selection to correspond to people's everyday experiences with the world, which illustrates an underlying cognitive linguistic premise that language is by and large both a reflection and product of our everyday interactions with the real world. Nevertheless, cognitive process and construction are complicated, which raises more questions of whether a semantic device or grammar use can be considered to be purely cognitive in nature. The book and the author's previous book on cognitive semantics in commercial discourses aim to help readers and researchers become aware of the meaning implications that have led the discourse writers to choose the lexis and grammars, and then to wrap linguistic applications. As cognitive operations are more often than not involved in the unravelling of the meaning of non-literal uses of language, the author has outlined and critically reviewed the most representative figurative uses of language and grammatical applications in discourses in the literature, and analysed their functions and construal meanings in authentic promotional and commercial texts. The author has illustrated that the meanings of cognitive expressions should be interpreted by integrating cognitive semantics and grammar elements, such as metonymy in point of view, stimulus in moves and modal verbs in grounding and their locations in syntax and discourses.

Cognition is a very complex internalization process that takes into account both internal and external aspects. This process embodies a complex system and a huge project of personalization, naturalization, ethnicization and knowledge construction, and there is still much room for research on how the limited cognition of the individual self can become a manifestation of absolute knowledge, such as how the individual's linguistic cognition is reflected in the outreach discourse. The cognitive exploration and logical construction of discourse strategies, which involve discourse constructions, syntax, lexical items and grammar in the structure of language, is a very popular area of research in applied linguistics, but much work is still needed to put them into empirical studies and cross-cultural contexts.

References

Abuczki, A. (2009). The use of metaphors in advertising: A case study and critical discourse analysis of advertisements in cosmopolitan. *Argumentum*, 5: 18-24.

Abutalebi, J. & Clahsen, H. (2015). Bilingualism, cognition, and aging. *Bilingualism: Language and Cognition*, 18(1): 1-2.

Afros, E. & Schryer, C. F. (2009). Promotional (meta)discourse in research articles in language and literary studies. *English for Specific Purposes*, 28(1): 58-68.

Al-Sharafi, A. (2004). *Textual Metonymy: A Semiotic Approach*. Hampshire: Palgrave Macmillan.

Andrea, M. (2004). *Prison Discourse: Language as a Means of Control and Resistance*. New York: Palgrave Macmillan.

Aski, J. M. (2001). Prototype categorization and phonological split. *Diachronica*, 18(2): 205-239.

Babbie, E. (2014). *The Basics of Social Research* (6th edn.). Belmont: Wadsworth Cengage.

Barnden, J. A. (2010). Metaphor and metonymy: Making their connections more slippery. *Cognitive Linguistics*, 21(1): 1-34.

Berg, B. & Lune, H. (2016). *Qualitative Research Methods for the Social Sciences* (9th edn.). London: Pearson.

Bhatia, V. K. (1993). *Analysing Genre: Language Use in Professional Settings*. London/New York: Longman.

Bhatia, V. K. (2004). *Worlds of Written Discourse: A Genre-based View*. Cornwall: Continuum.

Bhatia, V. K. (2005). Generic patterns in promotional discourse. In H. Halmari & T. Virtanen (Eds.), *Persuasion across Genres: A Linguistic Approach* (pp.213-225). Amsterdam: John Benjamins Publishing Company.

Bhatia, V. K. (2008). Genre analysis, ESP and professional practice. *English for Specific Purposes, 27*(2): 161-174.

Biber, D. & Zhang, M. (2018). Expressing evaluation without grammatical stance: Informational persuasion on the web. *Corpora, 13*(1): 97-123.

Bourdieu, P. (1991). *Language and Symbolic Power*. Cambridge: Cambridge University Press.

Boye, K. (2001). The force-dynamic core meaning of Danish modal verbs. *Acta Linguistica Hafniensia, 33*(1): 19-66.

Breeze, R. (2013). *Corporate Discourse*. London: Bloomsbury.

Brisard, F. (2002). *Grounding: The Epistemic Footing of Deixis and Reference*. Berlin: Mouton de Gruyter.

Broccias, C. (2021). *Cognitive grammar*. In X. Wen & J. R. Taylor (Eds.), *The Routledge Handbook of Cognitive Linguistics* (pp.30-42). New York: Routledge.

Bybee, J. L. (1985). *Morphology: A Study of the Relation between the Meaning and Form*. Amsterdam: John Benjamins Publishing Company.

Bybee, J. L. & Fleischman, S. (Eds.) (1995). *Modality in Grammar and Discourse*. Amsterdam: John Benjamins Publishing Company.

Bybee, J. L., Perkins, R. & Pagliuca, W. (1994). *The Evolution of Grammar: Tense, Aspect, and Modality in the Languages of the World*. Chicago: University of Chicago Press.

Caballero, R. (2009). Cutting across the senses: Imagery in winespeak and audiovisual promotion. In C. Forceville & E. Urios-Aparisi (Eds.), *Multimodal Metaphor* (pp.73-94). Berlin: Mouton de Gruyter.

Cap, P. (2006). *Legitimization in Political Discourse*. Newcastle: Cambridge Scholars Publishing.

Carter-Thomas, S. & Rowley-Jolivet, E. (2008). If-conditionals in medical discourse: From theory to disciplinary practice. *Journal of English for Academic Purposes, 7*(3): 191-205.

Charteris-Black, J. & Ennis, T. (2001). A comparative study of metaphor in Spanish and English financial reporting. *English for Specific Purposes, 20*(3): 249-266.

Charteris-Black, J. & Musolff, A. (2003). "Battered hero" or "innocent victim"? A comparative study of metaphors for euro trading in British and German financial reporting. *English for Specific Purposes, 22*(2): 153-176.

Chatterjee, A. (2010). Disembodying cognition. *Language and Cognition, 2*(1): 79-116.

Chaudhary, A. (2001). International news selection: A comparative analysis of negative news in *the Washington Post* and the *Daily Times* of Nigeria. *The Howard Journal of Communications, 12*(4): 241-254.

Chen, S. (2016). Selling the environment: Green marketing discourse in China's automobile advertising. *Discourse, Context & Media, 12*(C): 11-19.

Cheng, L. Y. & Yang, W. H. (2017). A contrastive discoursal study of cognitive frames in Chinese and American smog reports. *Journal of Guangdong University of Foreign Studies,* (1): 5-10. [程林燕，杨文慧. (2017). 中美雾霾报道的跨文化语篇认知构架探析. 广东外语外贸大学学报，(1)：5-10.]

Cheung, M. (2008). "Click here": The impact of new media on the encoding of persuasive messages in direct marketing. *Discourse Studies, 10* (2): 161-189.

Cheung, M. (2011). Sales promotion communication in Chinese and English: A thematic analysis. *Journal of Pragmatics, 43*(4): 1061-1079.

Chilton, P. (2004). *Analysing Political Discourse: Theory and Practice.* London: Routledge.

Chung, S. (2008). Cross-linguistic comparisons of the MARKET metaphors. *Corpus Linguistics and Linguistic Theory, 4*(2): 141-175.

Coates, J. (1985). *The Semantics of the Modal Auxiliaries.* London: Croom Helm.

Conko, G. (2011). Hidden truth: The perils and protection of off-label drug and medical device promotion. *Health Matrix: Journal of Law-Medicine, 21*(1): 149-187.

Connor, R. J. (1987). Sample Size for testing differences in proportions for the paired-sample design. *Biometrics, 43*(1): 207-211.

Croft, W. (1993). The role of domains in the interpretation of metaphors and metonymies. *Cognitive Linguistics, 4*(4): 335-370.

Croft, W. (1998). Linguistic evidence and mental representations. *Cognitive Linguistics, 9*(2): 151-174.

Croft, W. (2002). The role of domains in the interpretation of metaphors and metonymies. In R. Dirven & R. Porings (Eds.), *Metaphor and Metonymy in Comparison and Contrast* (pp.161-205). Berlin: Mouton de Gruyter.

Croft, W. & Cruse, D. (2004). *Cognitive Linguistics*. Cambridge: Cambridge University Press.

Dancygier, B. & Sanders, J. (2010). Textual choices and discourse genres: What cognitive linguistics reveals about form and meaning. *English Text Construction, 3*(2): 321-327.

Dancygier, B. & Sweetser, E. (2012). *Viewpoint in Language: A Multimodal Perspective*. Cambridge: Cambridge University Press.

De Beaugrande, R. A. & Dressler, W. (1981). *Introduction to Text Linguistics*. London: Longman.

Deetz, S. (1982). Critical interpretive research in organizational communication. *The Western Journal of Speech Communication, 46*(2): 131-149.

Desmet, K., Ortuño-Ortin, I. & Wacziarg, R. (2016). Linguistic cleavages and economic development. In V. Ginsburgh & S. Weber (Eds.), *The Palgrave Handbook of Economic and Language* (pp.425-446). London: Palgrave Macmillan.

Dirven, R. & Verspoor, M. (2004). *Cognitive Exploration of Language and Linguistics: Cognitive Linguistics in Practice* (2nd edn.). Amsterdam/ Philadelphia: John Benjamins Publishing Company.

Dirven, R., Wolf, H. G. & Polzenhagen, F. (2012). Cognitive linguistics and cultural studies. In G. Dirk & C. Hubert (Eds.), *The Oxford Handbook of Cognitive Linguistics* (pp.1203-1221). New York: Oxford University Press.

Drew, P. & Heritage, J. (1992). Analyzing talk at work: An introduction. In P. Drew & J. Heritage (Eds.), *Talk at Work: Interaction in Institutional Setting* (pp.3-65). Cambridge: Cambridge University Press.

Eggington, W. G. (1987). Written Academic Discourse in Korean: Implications for Effective Communication. In U. Connor & R. B. Kaplan (Eds.), *Writing across Languages: Analysis of L2 Text* (pp.153-168). Reading, MA: Addison-Wesley.

Entman, R. (1993). Framing: Toward clarification of a fractured paradigm. *Journal of Communication, 43*(4): 51-58.

Erjavec, K. (2004). Beyond advertising and journalism: Hybrid promotional news discourse. *Discourse & Society, 15*(5): 553-578.

Evans, V. & Green, M. (2006). *Cognitive Linguistics: An Introduction*.

Edinburgh: Edinburgh University Press.

Fairclough, N. (1992). *Discourse and Social Change.* Cambridge: Polity Press.

Fairclough, N. (1995). *Critical Discourse Analysis: The Critical Study of Language.* London: Longman.

Fairclough, N. (2003). *Analysing Discourse: Textual Analysis for Social Research.* London: Routledge.

Fauconnier, G. & Turner, M. (1996). Blending as a central process in grammar. In A. Goldberg (Ed.), *Conceptual Structure, Discourse, and Language* (pp.113-129). Stanford: Cambridge University Press.

Fauconnier, G. & Turner, M. (1998). Conceptual integration networks. *Cognitive Science, 22*(2): 133-187.

Fauconnier, G. & Turner, M. (2002). *The Way We Think: Conceptual Blending and the Mind's Hidden Complexities.* New York: Basic Books.

Fillmore, C. (1982). Frame semantics. In The Linguistic Society of Korea (Ed.), *Linguistics in the Morning Calm* (pp.111-122). Seoul: Hanshin Publishing Company.

Fillmore, C. (1985). Frames and the semantics of understanding. *Quaderni di Semantica, 6*(2): 222-254.

Fioramonte, A. & Vásquez, C. (2018). Multi-party talk in the medical encounter: Socio-pragmatic functions of family members' contributions in the treatment advice phase. *Journal of Pragmatics, 139*: 132-145.

Fowler, R. (1991). *Language in the News: Discourse and Ideology in the Press.* London: Routledge.

Fukuda, K. (2009). A comparative study of metaphors representing the US and Japanese economies. *Journal of Pragmatics, 41*(9): 1693-1702.

Gallardo, S. & Ferrari, L. (2010). How doctors view their health and professional practice: An appraisal analysis of medical discourse. *Journal of Pragmatics, 42*(12): 3172-3187.

Gärdenfors, P. (1995). *Conceptual Spaces as a Basis for Cognitive Semantics.* Netherlands: Springer.

Geeraerts, D. (2005). Lectal variation and empirical data in cognitive linguistics. In F. J. Ruiz De Mendoza & S. Peña Cervel (Eds.), *Cognitive Linguistics: Internal Dynamics and Interdisciplinary Interactions* (pp.163-189). Berlin: Mouton de Gruyter.

Geeraerts, D. (2006). Methodology in cognitive linguistics. In G. Kristiansen, M. Achard, R. Dirven & F. J. Ruiz De Mendoza (Eds.), *Cognitive Linguistics: Current Applications and Future Perspectives* (pp.21-49). New York: Mouton de Gruyter.

Geeraerts, D. (2010). Recontextualizing grammar: Underlying trends in thirty years of cognitive linguistics. In E. Tabakowska, M. Choinski & L. Wiraszka (Eds.), *Cognitive Linguistics in Action, from Theory to Application and Back* (pp.71-102). Berlin: Mouton de Gruyter.

Gibbs, R. (1999). Speaking and thinking with metonymy. In K. U. Panther & G. Radden (Eds.), *Metonymy in Language and Thought* (pp.61-90). Amsterdam: John Benjamins Publishing Company.

Given, L. M. (2008). *The SAGE Encyclopaedia of Qualitative Research Methods.* Los Angeles: SAGE Publications.

Givón, T. (1978). *Negation in Language: Pragmatics, Function, Ontology.* London: Academic Press.

Gogichev, C. (2016). Two categorization patterns in idiom semantics. *Pragmatics & Cognition, 23*(2): 343-358.

Goldberg, A. (2009). The nature of generalization in language. *Cognitive Linguistics, 20*(1): 93-127.

Gumperz, J. J. & Levinson, S. C. (Eds.) (1996). *Rethinking Linguistic Relativity.* Cambridge: Cambridge University Press.

Gunnarsson, B. L. (2006). Medical discourse: Sociohistorical construction. *Encyclopedia of Language and Linguistics,* (7): 709-717.

Guo, J. (2015). On the relationship between institutional discourse and language for specific purposes: Taking discourse community as the observation dimension. *Foreign Language Research,* (4): 49-52. [郭佳. (2015). 机构话语与专门用途语言的关系探析——以话语共同体为考察维度. 外语学刊, (4): 49-52.]

Habermas, J. (1984). *The Theory of Communicative Action: Reason and the Rationalization of Society (Vol. 1).* Boston: Beacon Press.

Halliday, M. A. K. (1994). *An Introduction to Functional Grammar* (2nd edn.). London: Edward Arnold.

Halliday, M. A. K. & Matthiessen, C. M. (2004). *An Introduction to Functional Grammar* (3rd edn.). London: Edward Arnold.

Handl, S. & Schmid, H. J. (2011). *Windows to the Mind: Metaphor, Metonymy and Conceptual Blending*. Berlin: Walter de Gruyter.

Harrison, C., Nuttall, L., Stockwell, P., et al. (2014). *Cognitive Grammar in Literature: Linguistic Approaches to Literature, vol. 17*. Amsterdam: John Benjamins Publishing Company.

Hart, C. (2014). *Discourse, Grammar and Ideology: Functional and Cognitive Perspectives*. London: Bloomsbury.

Hart, C. (2015). Viewpoint in linguistic discourse: Space and evaluation in news reports of political protests. *Critical Discourse Studies, 12*(3): 238-260.

Hartmann, R. R. K. (1980). *Contrastive Textology: Comparative Discourse Analysis in Applied Linguistics*. Heidelberg: Julius Groos Verlag.

Harvey, K. (2013). Medicalisation, pharmaceutical promotion and the Internet: A critical multimodal discourse analysis of hair loss websites. *Social Semiotics, 23*(5): 691-714.

Harwood, N. (2005). "Nowhere has anyone attempted ... In this article I aim to do just that": A corpus-based study of self-promotional: *I* and *we* in academic writing across four disciplines. *Journal of Pragmatics, 37*(8): 1207-1231.

Hatim, B. (2001). *Teaching and Researching Translation*. London: Pearson Education.

Heritage, J. & Drew, P. (1992). *Talk at Work: Interaction in Institutional Settings (Studies in Interactional Sociolinguistics)*. Cambridge: Cambridge University Press.

Holmes, J. & Stubbe, M. (2003). *Power and Politeness in the Workplace: A Sociolinguistic Analysis of Talk at Work*. London: Longman.

Holtgraves, T. M. & Yoshihisa, K. (2007). Language, meaning, and social cognition. *Personality and Social Psychology Review, 12*(1): 73-94.

Hou, S. T. & Zhang, Y. K. (2014). The study of main doctor-patient communication patterns and 6s extensions. *Medicine and Philosophy, 35*(1): 54-57. [侯胜田, 张永康. (2014). 主要医患沟通模式及 6s 延伸模式探讨. 医学与哲学, 35(1): 54-57.]

Hudson, R. (1984). *Word Grammar*. Oxford: Blackwell.

Hudson, R. (1988). Extraction and grammatical relation. *Lingua, 76*(2-3): 177-208.

Hudson, R. (2007). *Language Networks: The New Word Grammar.* Oxford: Oxford University Press.

Hudson, R. (2010). *An Introduction to Word Grammar.* Cambridge: Cambridge University Press.

Hyland, K. (1998). Hedging in scientific research articles. *English for Specific Purposes, 17*(3): 227-246.

Hyland, K. (2000). *Disciplinary Discourses: Social Interactions in Academic Writing.* Harlow: Longman.

Izquierdo, M. & Blanco, P. M. (2020). A multi-level contrastive analysis of promotional strategies in specialised discourse. *English for Specific Purposes, 58*: 43-57.

Jackendoff, R. (1990). *Semantic Structures: Current Studies in Linguistics.* Cambridge, Mass: The MIT Press.

Jakobson, R. (1971a). On linguistic aspects of translation. In R. Jakobson (Ed.), *Selected Writings 2: Word and Language* (pp.260-266). The Hague: Mouton de Gruyter.

Jakobson, R. (1971b). The metaphoric and metonymic poles. In R. Jakobson & M. Halle (Eds.), *Fundamentals of Language* (pp.90-96). The Hague: Mouton de Gruyter.

Jaworska, S. (2017). Metaphors we travel by: A corpus-assisted study of metaphors in promotional tourism discourse. *Metaphor and Symbol, 32*(3): 161-177.

Jiang, K. (2014). Review of corporate discourse. *English for Specific Purposes, 35*: 89-95.

Jing-Schmidt, Z. (2007). Negativity bias in language: A cognitive-affective model of emotive intensifiers. *Cognitive Linguistics, 18*(3): 417-443.

Johnson, M. (1987). *The Body in the Mind: The Bodily Basis of Meaning, Imagination, and Reason.* Chicago: The University of Chicago Press.

Johnson, M. (1993). *Moral Imagination: Implications of Cognitive Science for Ethics.* Chicago: University of Chicago Press.

Johnston, H. & Noakes, J. A. (2005). *Frames of Protest: Social Movements and the Framing Perspective.* Lanham: Rowman & Littlefield Publishers.

Joseph, J. & Droste, F. (1991). *Linguistic Theory and Grammatical Description.* Amsterdam: John Benjamins Publishing.

Kaplan, R. (1966). Cultural thought patterns in inter-cultural education. *Language Learning, 16*(1-2): 1-20.

Kaur, K., Arumugam, N. & Yunus, N. M. (2013). Beauty product advertisements: A critical discourse analysis. *Asian Social Science, 9*(3): 61-71.

Kimmel, M. (2011). Force dynamics in literary studies: A cognitive grammar approach. *Language and Literature, 20*(2): 121-135.

Kövecses, Z. (2006). *Language, Mind and Culture: A Practical Introduction.* Oxford: Oxford University Press.

Kövecses, Z. & Radden, G. (1998). Metonymy: Developing a cognitive linguistic view. *Cognitive Linguistics, 9*(1): 37-77.

Kreitzer, A. (2009). Multiple levels of schematization: A study in the conceptualization of space. *Cognitive Linguistics, 8*(4): 291-326.

Kristiansen, G. & Dirven, R. (2008). *Cognitive Sociolinguistics.* Berlin/Boston: Mouton De Gruyter.

Krzeszowski, T. P. (1989). Towards a typology of contrastive studies. In O. Wieslaw (Ed.), *Contrastive Pragmatics* (pp.55-72). Amsterdam: John Benjamins Publishing Company.

Lakoff, G. (1987). *Women, Fire, and Dangerous Things: What Categories Reveal about the Mind.* Chicago: University of Chicago Press.

Lakoff, G. (2002). *Moral Politics: How Liberals and Conservatives Think* (2nd edn.). Chicago: Chicago University Press.

Lakoff, G. & Johnson, M. (1980). *Metaphors We Live By.* Chicago: University of Chicago Press.

Lakoff, G. & Johnson, M. (1999). *Philosophy in the Flesh.* New York: Basic Books.

Lakoff, G. & Turner, M. (1989). *More than Cool Reason: A Field Guide to Poetic Metaphor.* Chicago: The University of Chicago Press.

Langacker, R. W. (1987a). *Foundations of Cognitive Grammar: Descriptive Application (Vol. 1).* Stanford: Stanford University Press.

Langacker, R. W. (1987b). Nouns and verbs. *Language, 63*: 53-94.

Langacker, R. W. (1991). *Foundations of Cognitive Grammar Vol. II: Descriptive Application.* Stanford: Stanford University Press.

Langacker, R. W. (1999). *Grammar and Conceptualization.* Berlin: Mouton de

Gruyter.

Langacker, R. W. (2001). The English present tense. *English Language and Linguistics*, 5(2): 251-272.

Langacker, R. W. (2002). *Grounding: The Epistemic Footing of Deixis and Reference*. Berlin/Boston: Mouton de Gruyter.

Langacker, R. W. (2004). *Foundations of Cognitive Grammar I*. Beijing: Peking University Press.

Langacker, R. W. (2008). *Cognitive Grammar: A Basic Introduction*. Oxford: Oxford University Press.

Lardiere, D. (2009). Some thoughts on the contrastive analysis of features in second language acquisition. *Second Language Research*, 25(2): 173-227.

Leech, G. (2003). Modality on the move: The English modal auxiliaries 1961-1992. In R. Facchinetti, M. Krug & F. Palmer (Eds.), *Modality in Contemporary English* (pp.223-240). Berlin/New York: Mouton de Gruyter.

Levinson, S. C. (1992). Activity type and language. In P. Drew & J. Heritage (Eds.), *Talk at Work: Interaction in Institutional Setting* (pp.66-101). Cambridge: Cambridge University Press.

Li, F. (2008). *An Introduction to Cognitive Linguistics*. Beijing: Peking University Press.

Li, T. X. (2013). *Discourse Coherence: A Cognitive Frame Approach*. Beijing: National Defence Industry Press. [李天贤. (2013). 认知框架视角下的语篇连贯研究. 北京：国防工业出版社.]

Li, Y. (2016). *Language Power and Social Harmony: A Study of the Social Effect of Institutional Discourse in China's Transformational Period*. Tianjin: Nankai University Press. [李艺. (2016). 语言权势与社会和谐——中国转型期机构话语社会效应研究. 天津：南开大学出版社.]

Li, Y. & Sun, C. X. (2016). Innovative development of "Internet plus medical treatment". *Macroeconomic Management*, (3): 33-35.

Li, Z. Z. (1998). Value orientation of contrastive discourse in English and Chinese texts. *Foreign Language Teaching and Research*, (1): 14-17. [李战子. (1998). 英汉语篇研究中对比话语的价值取向. 外语教学与研究，(1)：14-17.]

Li, Z. Z. (2001). Multiple interpersonal meanings of epistemic modality in academic discourse. *Foreign Language Teaching and Research*, (5): 353-358.

[李战子. (2001). 学术话语中认知型情态的多重人际意义. 外语教学与研究，(5)：353-358.]

Lim, F.V. (2004). Developing an integrative multi-semiotic model. In K.L. O'Halloran (ed.), *Multi-modal Discourse Analysis* (pp.220-246). London: Continuum.

Littlemore, J. (2015). *Metonymy: Hidden Shortcuts in Language, Thought and Communication.* Cambridge: Cambridge University Press.

Liu, L. H. (2008). Modal verbs analysis in media discourses. *Journal of Tianjin Foreign Studies University,* (5): 21-29. [刘立华. (2008). 媒体语篇中的情态动词分析. 天津外国语大学学报，(5)：21-29.]

Lu, G. Q. (1999). *A Contrastive Analysis of Semantic Structure in English and Chinese.* Shanghai: Fudan University Press. [陆国强. (1999). 英汉和汉英语义结构对比. 上海：复旦大学出版社.]

Lu, W. Z. & Lu, Y. (2006). The cognitive mechanism of discourse cohesion and coherence. *Foreign Language Education, 27*(1): 13-18. [卢卫中，路云. (2006). 语篇衔接与连贯的认知机制. 外语教学，27(1)：13-18.]

Lü, S. J. & Huang, P. (2015). The principle of goal direction and the study of institutional discourse. *Foreign Language Research,* (3): 62-65. [吕殊佳，黄萍. (2015). 语用目的原则与机构性话语研究. 外语学刊，(3)：62-65.]

Lü, S. X. (1982). *A Brief Introduction to Chinese Grammar.* Beijing: The Commercial Press. [吕叔湘. (1982). 中国文法要略. 北京：商务印书馆.]

Lyons, J. (1977). *Semantics.* Cambridge: Cambridge University Press.

Ma, B. S. (2002). A review of contrastive discourse in China: Its current situation and use for reference. *Foreign Languages and Their Teaching,* (10): 37-40. [马博森. (2002). 国内对比语篇研究：现状与借鉴. 外语与外语教学，(10)：37-40.]

Ma. Z. J., Liu, J. & Chen, H. Q. (2017). The prosodic feature of modal verbs in Chinese courtroom discourse and its interpersonal function. *Contemporary Rhetoric,* (6): 33-41. [马泽军，刘佳，陈海庆. (2017). 庭审话语中情态动词的韵律特征及其人际功能实现.当代修辞学，(6)：33-41.]

Maalej, A. Z. & Yu, N. (2011). Introduction: Embodiment via body parts. In Z. Maalej & N. Yu (Eds.), *Embodiment via Body Parts: Studies from Various Languages and Cultures* (pp.1-20). Amsterdam: John Benjamins Publishing Company.

Maat, H. P. (2007). How promotional language in press releases is dealt with by journalists: Genre mixing or genre conflict? *The Journal of Business Communication, 44*(1): 59-95.

Mahon, J. E. (1999). Getting your sources right. In L. Cameron & G. Low (Eds.), *Researching and Applying Metaphor* (pp.69-80). Cambridge: Cambridge University Press.

Martin, J. E. (1992). *Towards a Theory of Text for Contrastive Rhetoric: An Introduction to Issues of Text for Students and Practitioners of Contrastive Rhetoric.* New York: Peter Lang.

Mashak, S. P., Pazhakh, A. & Hayati, A. (2012). A comparative study on basic emotion conceptual metaphors in English and Persian literary texts. *International Education Studies, 5*(1): 200-207.

Mayr, A. (2004). Doing "institutional talk": The story of a mock negotiation. *Journal of Pragmatics, 36*(7): 1231-1260.

Miao, X. W. (2006). Advances and frontiers of discourse analysis. *Foreign Language Research,* (1): 44-49. [苗兴伟. (2006). 语篇分析的进展与前沿. 外语学刊, (1)：44-49.]

Minsky, M. (1975). A framework for representing knowledge. In P. H. Winston (Ed.), *The Psychology of Computer Vision* (pp.211-277). New York: McGraw-Hill.

Mirador, J. F. (2000). A move analysis of written feedback in higher education. *RELC Journal, 31* (1): 45-60.

Misir, H. & Işik-Güler, H. (2022). "Be a better version of you!": A corpus-driven critical discourse analysis of MOOC platforms' marketing communication. *Linguistics and Education, 69*: 1-12.

Moynihan, R., Heath, I. & Henry, D. (2002). Selling sickness: the pharmaceutical industry and disease mongering. *BMJ, 324*(7342): 886–891.

Nisbett, R. E. & Miyamoto, Y. (2005). The influence of culture: Holistic versus analytic perception. *Trends in Cognitive Sciences, 9*: 467-473.

Nwogu, K. N. (1991). Structure of science popularizations: A genre-analysis approach to the schema of popularized medical texts. *English for Specific Purposes, 10*(2): 111-123.

Palmer, F. R. (1987). *The English Verb* (2nd edn.). London/New York: Longman.

Palmer, F. R. (1990). *Modality and the English Modals* (2nd edn.). London/New York: Longman.

Palmer, F. R. (2001). *Mood and Modality*. Cambridge: Cambridge University Press.

Pankow, C. (1992). *Sign, Language and Ritual: Contrastive Discourse Analysis of East German and Soviet TV News*. Abo: Abo Akademis Forlag.

Panther, K. U. & Thornburg, L. (1998). A Cognitive approach to inferencing in conversation. *Journal of Pragmatics, 30*(6): 755-769.

Panther, K. U. & Thornburg, L. (1999). The potentiality for actuality metonymy in English and Hungarian. In K. U. Panther & G. Radden (Eds.), *Metonymy in Language and Thought* (pp.333-360). Amsterdam: John Benjamins Publishing Company.

Panther, K. U. & Thornburg, L. (2007). Metonymy. In D. Geeraerts & H. Cuyckens (Eds.), *The Oxford Handbook of Cognitive Linguistics* (pp.236-316). Oxford: Oxford University Press.

Peirsman, Y. & Geeraerts, D. (2006). Metonymy as a prototypical category. *Cognitive Linguistics, 17*(3): 269-316.

Peng, K. & Nisbett, R. E. (1999). Culture, dialectics, and reasoning about contradiction. *American Psychologist, 54*(9): 741-754.

Peng, L. Z. (2007).*Modality in Modern Mandarin*. Beijing: China Social Sciences Press. [彭利贞. (2007). 现代汉语情态研究. 北京：中国社会科学出版社.]

Peng, Y. & Bai, J. H. (2007). A cognitive contrastive approach to ANGER neologisms in Chinese and English. *Journal of Foreign Languages*, (6): 32-38. [彭懿, 白解红. (2007). 汉英 "愤怒" 情感新词的认知对比研究. 外国语, (6)：32-38.]

Perkins, M. R. (1983). *Modal Expressions in English*. London: Pinter.

Pilnick, A. & Dingwall, R. (2001). Research directions in genetic counselling: A review of the literature. *Patient Education Counseling, 44*(2): 95-105.

Preminger, A. & Brogan, T. (1993). *The New Princeton Encyclopedia of Poetry and Poetics*. Princeton: Princeton University Press.

Qian, Y. (1983). A comparison of some cohesive devices in English and Chinese. *Journal of Foreign Languages,* (1): 19-26. [钱瑗. (1983). 英汉衔接手段之比较. 外国语(上海外国语大学学报)，(1)：19-26.]

Quirk, R., Greenbaum, S., Leech, G., et al. (1985). *A Comprehensive Grammar of the English Language*. London/New York: Longman.

Radden, G. & Dirven, R. (2007). *Cognitive English Grammar*. Amsterdam: John Benjamins Publishing Company.

Radden, G. & Kövecses, Z. (1999). Towards a theory of metonymy. In K. U. Panther & G. Radden (Eds.), *Metonymy in Language and Thought* (pp.91-120). Amsterdam: John Benjamins Publishing Company.

Radden, G. & Kövecses, Z. (2007). Towards theory of metonymy. In V. Evans, B. Bergen & J. Zinken (Eds.), *The Cognitive Linguistics Reader* (pp.335-359). London: Equinox.

Ren, K. & Wang, Z. H. (2017). A comparative study of Chinese and English modality in political news discourse: A perspective of systemic functional linguistics. *Contemporary Foreign Languages Studies*, (2): 20-26. [任凯，王振华. (2017). 系统功能语言学视角下的英汉情态对比研究——以政治新闻语篇为例. 当代外语研究，(2)：20-26.]

Richardson, A. W. (2002). Engineering philosophy of science: American pragmatism and logical empiricism in the 1930s. *Philosophy of Science*, 69(S3): 36-47.

Rucker, D., Petty, R. & Briñol, P. (2008). What's in a frame anyway?: A meta-cognitive analysis of the impact of one versus two sided message framing on attitude certainty. *Journal of Consumer Psychology*, 18(2): 137-149.

Ruffolo, I. (2015). The greening of hotels in the UK and Italy: A cross-cultural study of the promotion of environmental sustainability of comparable corpora of hotel websites. *Procedia-Social and Behavioral Sciences*, 198: 397-408.

Ruiz de Mendoza, F. J. & Baicchi, A. (2007). Illocutionary constructions: Cognitive motivation and linguistic realization. In I. Kecskes & L. Horn (Eds.), *Explorations in Pragmatics: Linguistic, Cognitive, and Intercultural Aspects* (pp.95-128). Berlin/New York: Mouton de Gruyter.

Ruiz de Mendoza, F. J. & Galera, A. (2014). *Cognitive Modeling: A Linguistic Perspective*. Amsterdam: John Benjamins Publishing Company.

Ruiz de Mendoza, F. J. & Mairal, R. (2008). Levels of description and constraining factors in meaning construction: an introduction to the lexical constructional model. *Folia Linguistica, 42*(2): 355-400.

Ruiz de Mendoza, F. J. & Mairal, R. (2011). Constrains on syntactic alternation: lexical-constructional subsumption in the Lexical Construction Model. In P. Guerrero (Ed.), *Morphosyntactic Alternations in English: Functional and Cognitive Perspectives* (pp.62-82). London, UK & Oakville, CT: Equinox.

Semino, E. (2002). A sturdy baby or a derailing train? Metaphorical representations of the euro in British and Italian newspapers. *TEXT, 22*(1): 107-139.

Seto, K. (1999). Distinguishing metonymy from synecdoche. In K. U. Panther & G. Radden (Eds.), *Metonymy in Language and Thought* (pp.91-120). Amsterdam: John Benjamins Publishing Company.

Schiffrin, D., Tannen, D. & Hamilton, H. E. (Eds.) (2001). *The Handbook of Discourse Analysis*. London: Blackwell.

Schubert, C. (2014). Cognitive categorization and prototypicality as persuasive strategies: Presidential rhetoric in the USA. *Journal of Language and Politics, 13*(2): 313-335.

Schumann, J. H. (1994). Where is cognition? Emotion and cognition in second language acquisition. *Studies in Second Language Acquisition, 16*(2): 231-242.

Scollon, R. & Scollon, S. (1995). *Intercultural Communication: A Discourse Approach*. Malden, Mass: Blackwell.

Scollon, R. & Scollon, S. (2000). *Intercultural Communication*. London: Blackwell.

Scollon, R., Scollon, S. & Kirkpatrick, A. (2000). *Contrastive Discourse in Chinese and English: A Critical Appraisal*. Beijing: Foreign Language Teaching and Research Press.

Semino, E. & Culpeper, J. (Eds.) (2002). *Cognitive Stylistics: Language and Cognition in Text Analysis*. Amsterdam: John Benjamins Publishing Company.

Sharafi, A. & Gabbar, A. (2004). *Textual Metonymy: A Semiotic Approach*. New York: Palgrave Macmillan.

Shields, P. & Rangarajan, N. (2013). *A Playbook for Research Methods: Integrating Conceptual Frameworks and Project Management*. Stillwater: New Forums Press.

Shu, D. F. (2008). *Cognitive Semantics*. Shanghai: Shanghai Foreign Language

Education Press.

Silverman, D. (1997). *Discourses of Counselling: HIV Counselling as Social Interaction*. London: Sage.

Sinclair, J. M. & Coulthard, R. M. (1975). *Towards an Analysis of Discourse*. Oxford: Oxford University Press.

Singh, R. & Kachroo, B. (1987). Textual cohesion in Hindi: A comparative study. *ITL-International Journal of Applied Linguistics, 76* (1): 1-24.

Sinha, C. (2021). Culture in language and cognition. In X. Wen & J. R. Taylor (Eds.), *The Routledge Handbook of Cognitive Linguistics* (pp.387-409). New York: Routledge.

Sinha, C. & Jensen de López, K. (2000). Language, culture and the embodiment of spatial cognition. *Cognitive Linguistics, 11*(1-2): 17-41.

Snow, D. A., Rochford, E. B., Worden, S. K., et al. (1986). Frame alignment processes, micromobilization, and movement participation. *American Sociological Review, 51*(4): 464–481.

Snow, D. A. & Benford, R. D. (1992). Master frames and cycles of protest. In A. D. Morris & C. Mueller (Eds.), *Frontiers in Social Movement Theory* (pp.133-155). New Haven, CT: Yale University Press.

Stibel, J. M. (2006). Categorization and technology innovation. *Pragmatics & Cognition, 14*(2): 343-355.

Stockwell, P. (2009). *Texture: A Cognitive Aesthetics of Reading*. Edinburgh: Edinburgh University Press.

Suau-Jiménez, F. (2020). Closeness and distance through the agentive authorial voice: Construing credibility in promotional discourse. *International Journal of English Studies, 20*(1): 73-92.

Sulaiman, M. Z. (2014). Translating the style of tourism promotional discourse: A cross cultural journey into stylescapes. *Procedia-Social and Behavioral Sciences, 118*: 503-510.

Swales, J. (1990). *Genre Analysis: English in Academic and Research Settings*. Cambridge: Cambridge University Press.

Swales, J. (2004). *Research Genres: Explorations and Applications*. Cambridge: Cambridge University Press.

Sweetser, E. (1990). *From Etymology to Pragmatics: Metaphorical and Cultural Aspects of Semantic Structure*. Cambridge: Cambridge University Press.

Talmy, L. (1985). Lexicalization patterns: Semantic structure in lexical forms. In T. Shopen (Ed.). *Language Typology and Syntactic Description* (pp.57-149). *Vol. III: Grammatical Categories and the Lexicon*. Cambridge: Cambridge University Press.

Talmy, L. (1988). Force dynamics in language and cognition. *Cognitive Science, 12*(1): 49-100.

Talmy, L. (2000). *Toward a Cognitive Semantics*. Cambridge: MIT Press.

Taylor, J. (1995). *Linguistic Categorization: Prototypes in Linguistic Theory* (2nd edn.). Oxford: Oxford University Press.

Thornborrow, J. (2002). *Power Talk: Language and Interaction in Institutional Discourse*. Harlow: Longman.

Trabant, J. (2000). How relativistic are Humboldt's "Weltansichten"? In M. Pütz & M. Verspoor (Eds.), *Explorations in Linguistic Relativity* (pp.25-44). Amsterdam: John Benjamins Publishing Company.

Turner, M. (1991). Conceptual blending and the mind's hidden complexities. In D. Gentner & A. Stevens (Eds.), *Mental Models* (pp.257-294). Mahwah: Lawrence Erlbaum Associates.

Ullmann, S. (1962). *Semantics: An Introduction to the Science of Meaning*. Oxford: Blackwell.

Ungerer, F. & Schmid, H. J. (2006). *An Introduction to Cognitive Linguistics*. London/New York: Longman.

Upton, T. & Cohen, M. (2009). An approach to corpus-based discourse analysis: The move analysis as example. *Discourse Studies, 11*(5): 585-605.

van Dijk, T. A. (1977). *Text and Context: Explorations in the Semantics and Pragmatics of Discourse*. London/New York: Longman.

van Dijk, T. A. (1980). *Macrostructures: An Interdisciplinary Study of Global Structures in Discourse, Interaction, and Cognition*. Mahwah: Lawrence Erlbaum Associates.

van Dijk, T. A. (1985). Semantic discourse analysis. In T. A. van Dijk (Ed.), *Handbook of Discourse Analysis* (pp.103-112). London: Academic Press.

van Dijk, T. A. (1988). *News as Discourse*. Hillsdale, NJ: Erlbaum.

van Dijk, T. A. (1998). *Ideology: A Multidisciplinary Approach*. London: Sage Publication.

van Dijk, T. A. (2006). Discourse, context and cognition. *Discourse Study, 8*(1):

159-177.

van Dijk, T. A. (2008). *Discourse and Power*. New York: Palgrave Macmillan.

Vergaro, C. (2004). Discourse strategies of Italian and English sales promotion letters. *English for Specific Purposes, 23*(2): 181-207.

Virtanen, T. (2004). *Approaches to Cognition through Text and Discourse*. Berlin: Walter de Gruyter.

Wallmach, K. & Kruger, A. (1999). "Putting a sock on it": A contrastive analysis of problem-solving translation strategies between African and European languages. *South African Journal of African Languages, 19*(4): 276-289.

Wang, H., Runtsova, T. & Chen, H. (2013). Economy is an organism: A comparative study of metaphor in English and Russian economic discourse. *Text & Talk, 33*(2): 259-288.

Wang, H. J. & Feng, Y. Y. (2017). Effect of "Internet + healthcare" on the traditional healthcare service delivery mode and physician-patient relationship and the suggested countermeasures. *Chinese General Practice, 20*(25): 3191-3194. [王慧君, 冯跃林. (2017). "互联网+医疗"对医疗服务模式和医患关系的影响及应对分析. 中国全科医学, 20(25): 3191-3194.]

Wang, H. L. & Guo, J. R. (2006). Genre analysis and promotional discourses. *Foreign Language Education, 27*(4): 32-37. [王宏俐, 郭继荣. (2006). 体裁分析与商务促销类语篇. 外语教学, 27(4): 32-37.]

Wang, M. X. & Li, J. (1993). A survey about Chinese students' English discourse thinking mode. *Foreign Language Teaching and Research,* (4): 59-64. [王墨希, 李津. (1993). 中国学生英语语篇思维模式调查. 外语教学与研究, (4): 59-64.]

Wang, Y. (2002). Cognitive semantics. *Journal of Sichuan International Studies University, 18*(2): 58-62. [王寅. (2002). 认知语义学. 四川外国语大学学报, 18(2): 58-62.]

Wang, Y. (2006). *Cognitive Linguistics*. Shanghai: Shanghai Foreign Language Education Press. [王寅. (2006). 认知语言学. 上海: 上海外语教育出版社.]

Wardhaugh, R. & Fuller, J. M. (2015). *An Introduction to Sociolinguistics*. New Jersey: Blackwell.

Wen, X. (1999). A review of cognitive linguistics research abroad. *Journal of*

Foreign Languages, (1): 35-41. [文旭. (1999). 国外认知语言学研究综观. 外国语(上海外国语大学学报)，(1)：35-41.]

Wen, X. (2002). On the objectives, principles, and methodology of cognitive linguistics. *Foreign Language Teaching and Research,* (2): 90-97. ［文旭. (2002). 认知语言学的研究目标、原则和方法. 外语教学与研究，(2)：90-97.]

Wen, X. (2014). *Cognitive Foundation of Language.* Beijing: Science Press. [文旭. (2014). 语言的认知基础. 北京：科学出版社.]

Wilce, J. (2009). Medical discourse. *Annual Review of Anthropology, 38*: 199-215.

William-Jones, B. (2006). Be ready against cancer now: direct-to-consumer advertising for genetic testing. *New Genetics and Society, 25*(1): 89-107.

Wodak, R. (1996). *Disorders of Discourse.* London: Longman.

Wu, S. X. & Chen, W. Z. (2004). Development of category theory and its contributions to cognitive linguistics. *Journal of Foreign Languages,* (4): 34-40. [吴世雄，陈维振. (2004). 范畴理论的发展及其对认知语言学的贡献. 外国语，(4)：34-40.]

Xiong, T. (2012). Discourse and marketization of higher education in China: The genre of advertisements for academic posts. *Discourse & Society, 23*(3): 318-337.

Xiong, T. & Li, Q. N. (2020). Interdiscursivity and promotional discourse: A corpus-assisted genre analysis of about us texts on Chinese university websites. *Chinese Journal of Applied Linguistics, 43*(4): 397-416, 525. [熊涛，李秋娜. (2020). 话语间性和推广话语：语料库辅助的中国大学网站简介体裁分析. 中国应用语言学，43(4)：397-416，525.]

Xiong, X. L. (1999). *An Introduction to Cognitive Pragmatics.* Shanghai: Shanghai Foreign Language Education Press. [熊学亮. (1999). 认知语用学概论. 上海：上海外语教育出版社.]

Xu, J. (2005). A contrastive study of interpersonal function between the Chinese and English versions of The Scholar. *Journal of PLA University of Foreign Languages,* (6): 14-17. [徐珺. (2005).《儒林外史》汉英语篇之人际功能对比研究. 解放军外国语学院学报，(6)：14-17.]

Xu, L. S. (2004). On cross-cultural contrastive discourse analysis. *Journal of Zhejiang University (Humanities and Social Sciences),* (4): 110-117. [许力生.

(2004). 语篇跨文化对比的问题分析. 浙江大学学报(人文社会科学版), (4)：110-117.]

Xu, Y. L. (1992). *An Introduction to Contrastive Linguistics.* Shanghai：Shanghai Foreign Language Education Press. [许余龙. (1992). 对比语言学概论. 上海：上海外语教育出版社.]

Yan, T. Q. (2021). A cognitive construal approach to the narration in the Handmaid's tale. *Foreign Language and Literature Research, 7*(1): 49-56. [严天欣. (2021). 识解理论视角下《使女的故事》的叙事研究. 外国语文研究，7(1)：49-56.]

Yang, W. H. (2009). On the intercultural pragmatic differences and stereotype: A discourse study of thematic structure in communication. *Foreign Languages and Literature, 25*(3): 93-99. [杨文慧. (2009). 从主位结构的运用看跨文化语用差异和语用定势. 外国语文，25(3)：93-99.]

Yang, W. H. (2020). *A Cross-cultural Study of Commercial Media Discourses: From the Perspective of Cognitive Semantics.* Berlin: Springer.

Yang, W. H. (2023). On cognitive S-T-A models in news discourses of Sino-American trade negotiations. *Modern Foreign Language, 46*(3): 332-344. [杨文慧. (2023). 中美贸易谈判新闻语篇中语法空间认知模式研究. 现代外语，46(3)：332-344.]

Yang, W. H., Cheng, L. Y. & Zhen, K. Y. (2020). Cognitive analysis of the "discourse stances" in English news reports on smog in China and America. *International Journal of English Linguistics, 10*(4): 1-14.

Yang, W. H., Liang, Q. C. & Zhen, K. Y. (2016). A discourse study of cognitive frame construction of "China" in American economic news. *English Linguistic Research, 5*(4): 7-24.

Yang, Y. & Dong, F. (2016). A cognitive discourse analysis of the "medicine is war" metaphor. *Foreign Language and Literature Research, 2*(5): 26-35.

Yu, F. Q. & Yue, C. (2011). Unpromotable medical income. *China Weekly,* (12): 39-40. [于芳倩, 岳辰. (2011). 推不动的医疗收入. 中国周刊, (12)：39-40.]

Yue, M. & Liu, H. T. (2011). Probability distribution of discourse relations based on a Chinese RST-annotated corpus. *Journal of Quantitative Linguistics, 18*(2): 107-121.

Zeng, X. Y. (2008). Six basic features of cognitive semantics. *Foreign Languages Research,* (5): 20-23.

Zhang, C. & Xu, C. (2017). Argument by multimodal metaphor as strategic maneuvering in video advertising: The case of the Lin Dan Commercial. *Journal of Argumentation in Context*, 6(3): 359-380.

Zhang, H. & Lu, W. Z. (2010). *Cognitive Metonymy*. Shanghai: Shanghai Foreign Language Education Press. [张辉, 卢卫忠. (2010). 认知转喻. 上海：上海外语教育出版社.]

Zhang, H. & Luo, Y. L. (2017). A critical cognitive analysis of strategic intelligence discourse: A perspective from cognitive grammar. *Foreign Languages Research, 34*(6): 4-10, 112. [张辉, 罗一丽. (2017). 战略情报话语的批评认知分析——认知语法的视角. 外语研究，34(6)：4-10，112.]

Zhang, H. & Zhang, T. W. (2012). Cognitive metonymy approach to critical discourse analysis. *Foreign Language and Literature,* (3): 41-46. [张辉，张天伟. (2012). 批评话语分析的认知转喻视角研究. 外国语文，(3)：41-46.]

Zhang, J. L. (2006). An English-Chinese contrastive study on polysemous networks of Heart. *Journal of Zhejiang University, 36*(3): 161-168. [张建理. (2006). 英汉"心"的多义网络对比. 浙江大学学报，36(3)：161-168.]

Zhang, W., Speelman, D. & Geeraerts, D. (2015). Cross-linguistic variation in metonymies for PERSON: A Chinese-English contrastive study. *Review of Cognitive Linguistics. Published under the Auspices of the Spanish Cognitive Linguistics Association, 13*(1): 220-256.

Zhao, J. Y. & Feng, Y. (2012). Modal resources in commercial advertising discourse. *Journal of Northeast Normal University (Philosophy and Social Sciences),* (2): 222-223. [赵金宇，冯彦. (2012). 商业广告语篇中的情态资源. 东北师大学报(哲学社会科学版)，(2)：222-223.]

Zhao, Y. F. (2002). *An Introduction to Cognitive Linguistics*. Shanghai: Shanghai Foreign Language Education Press. [赵艳芳. (2002). 认知语言学概论. 上海：上海外语教育出版社.]

Zhu, G. M. (2005). Modality and Chinese modal verbs. *Shandong Foreign Languages Teaching Journal,* (2): 17-21. [朱冠明. (2005). 情态与汉语情态动词. 山东外语教学，(2)：17-21.]